Almost Home

How I Lost My Mother Without Losing My Mind:
A Faith Journey

Teresa M. Norris

Husky Trail Press LLC

Dedication

*This book is dedicated to my mother,
Mary S. Christo,
who taught me faith–not only by her life,
but through her death as well.*

Contents

Introduction

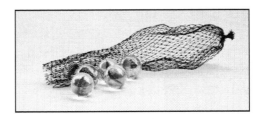

The Beginning

When my mother lost her marbles, she saw it coming. "Everyone thinks I'm losing my marbles," she'd complain to me on the phone. I, her only daughter, would try to reassure her, hiding from her the realization that I too had come upon over the last several months: Dementia was taking its toll. She was not the same.

Striving to be the "cheerleader," I sent her a bag of marbles in the mail with a note reading: "The next time someone says, 'Mary, you're losing your marbles,' you can show them these and tell them you know exactly where they are." We both had a good laugh over that.

Unfortunately, it offered little comfort as time progressed.

As finding comfort became increasingly important, I tapped into what I always had: my faith in God and the gift He'd given me—writing.

As a first grade teacher, I would sometimes tell

my young students: Writing saves things. For me, as a middle-aged woman, I must add: Writing can save *you*. As I fought my way through an emotional minefield, watching my elderly mother slip away with dementia and death, my journal writing provided me with a cathartic means of dealing with a painful situation.

My writing both validated my feelings and vindicated me from the oppressive guilt that wove its way through my experiences with my mother while she was in a nursing home. She died almost two years to the day that she entered the home, and through those months there were many heart-wrenching visits.

Having kept a prayer journal for many years, my earlier accounts included in this book have been reconstructed from those pages. Later, when influenced by more specific "life-experience" writing, I wrote at greater length after each trip to the nursing home. Sitting down with my laptop computer, I allowed the words and feelings to flow. The process provided me with an outlet I sorely needed.

Though by definition very personal, this account is possibly universal. In being such, it seems I should at least attempt to share this story. If writing indeed "saves things," then reading what someone else has saved may evoke a shared experience. And sharing experiences is at least part of what defines our humanity. That the spiritual connection is also evident throughout my many musings is an important bonus. And God, ever faithful, is the bonus I believe we must eventually acknowledge in our lives.

The Book

The first several months of my mother's stay in the nursing home were recorded in part through my regular prayer journaling. For decades I have kept a journal where I "just talk to God," never expecting anyone else to read my entries. Since they provided needed records of what happened at the start of this story, I decided I had to include them. As I extracted the entries from the handwritten pages of my journal, two things struck me: The self-centeredness of my writing and the faithfulness of God. Considering the journal was always meant to be *my* recording of what mattered to me, it seemed less selfish and more understandable for it to have exactly that slant. As far as the "God thing?" Well, my journaling *was* set up as a conversation with God. No surprises there.

For the sake of consistency of "voice," I transcribed the journal additions into a more "I'm just talking to *myself*" mode, which is how the later essays were done. I also realized I should edit some of the journal entries at least to clarify places or people I might mention.

The essays differed from the journal entries in that each one was written to "stand alone," and I did expect others might read them. In both cases, however, they were my *personal reflections* given at the time events occurred. Throughout the entire book I have added some commentary to expand on or help clarify the context. Toward that end, I now offer some background information as well.

The Background

My parents lived all their married lives in Tiverton, RI and my older brother John and I were raised there. Ours was a close family with aunts and uncles living on the same street and family gatherings held in our backyard. My maternal grandmother, who lived at my godmother's house nearby, underscored our Portuguese heritage. Though she'd emigrated from the Azores as a teenager, she never learned to speak English. (This seemed to give the adults in my family an advantage over us kids: they'd just speak Portuguese when they didn't want us to know what was going on!)

Our Catholic church was just up the street and hosted the sacraments from baptisms to funerals for our family members. We attended church every Sunday, and there was a large framed photograph collage of my brother's and my First Communion on display at our house. I remember sitting on the couch with my mother as she read from a book on the lives of the saints, and I probably could recite my "Our Father" and "Hail Mary" before I knew my phone number.

The childhood my brother and I enjoyed was rich with family traditions, deep-rooted faith, and the innocence of simpler times. Our parents did their best in providing a loving, strict upbringing where we may at times have felt overprotected, but never neglected.

Our neighborhood was nestled along Narragansett Bay, though unfortunately oil tanks spoiled what had been a lovely scenic expanse when my mother grew up there. A two-room schoolhouse was just three blocks away, allowing me to walk to school until I finished fourth grade. After that I took the bus to the schools at the "top of the hill," still within a mile of my house. Since my town didn't have a high school at that time, I was later bussed out to schools in nearby Fall River, MA.

My mother cried when in the late 60's I headed off to college, a whole hour away at the University of RI. There I debated between pursuing a degree in journalism or child development. I chose the latter, thinking it more practical as I planned to marry and have children. (Obviously I had not caught up with the women's movement!)

In 1970 I did marry a young man from CT and we soon settled there. While I now lived a two-hour drive away from our parents, my brother had married earlier and built his house right behind our parents' home. While he might see them every day, I relied on visits back and forth and numerous phone conversations each week. Our faith connection persevered though, and my parents and I would go on retreats together and share "praise-the Lord-reports."

But time does have a way of changing things.

As our parents aged, roles were gradually reversed. The caring and the decisions became the children's to be made for the parents. My brother's proximity made him the obvious prime caretaker. However, he and I would consult regularly, and in time we had to face our inability to meet our parents' needs.

As our parents entered their mid-eighties, things really began to unravel. I remember when I realized my mother had a serious memory problem. I'd thought it unsettling enough that in phone conversations she'd ask the same question several

XIV

times. But the occasion that changed concern into fear was when she forgot I was going to my son's college graduation one May weekend in 1997. She would *never* forget something as important as that, and of course I'd been telling her of our plans for weeks.

When we had our usual Sunday night phone call and she asked me what we had done that weekend, I knew something was *wrong*. I knew that things would be changing and they would never be the same again. Her life journey, and with hers our family's, would now be taking a terrible turn. We were entering that time that must come when an elderly parent prepares to move on. Though "almost home," the path may be long and arduous.

Here begins the story of my mother's passing.

The Story

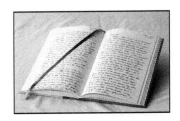

As I've said, my elderly parents were living in their own home in Rhode Island as they had for decades. My brother John built his house practically in their back yard, and through the early years they all enjoyed the closeness. Babysitting, family cookouts and the like were standard fare. My parents and I would visit back and forth from my home in central Connecticut and of course there were many phone calls connecting us. My phone conversations with my parents (usually my mom) also provided news on my brother and his own brood of four children.

John rarely called me himself, but in our parents' later years he sometimes needed to break some bad news to me. It got to a point, unfortunately, where my heart would stop just hearing his voice on the phone. He'd quickly tell me, "Everything's all right," if in fact it was. On this occasion, it wasn't.

Journal Entry: November 3, 2001

Well, they say when it rains, it pours. This morning my brother called to tell me our mom had fallen–not hurt–but was going to the hospital–and then? I was doing report cards–after waking up at 4:00 A.M. with a migraine. So, of course, the guilt and uncertainty kicked in. Should I drop what I'm doing and drive the two hours to RI to see them? Three or four phone calls later, I was told (after having already decided) I didn't need to go over there. Still, I feel guilty and not sure it was the right decision.

I spoke with my mom and dad on the phone and got mixed messages even there. I guess I'll have to wait and see. I did push to get my report cards done, so if things do get worse, at least that stress won't be added. Of course I don't mean to sound so self-centered. I feel mostly for my dad who must be missing my mom and wondering what will be next. Still, poor man, he's been through this before.

Guilt was always pulling at me when I'd get these kinds of calls. Living two hours away and teaching full time, I couldn't exactly just jump in my car and drive over there to check things out myself or lend the support I knew I could. Often, after deciding not to go, I'd jump every time the phone rang or constantly second-guess myself as to what decision I had made. If I'd lived ten hours away, or only ten minutes away, it would have been easier to decide such things and easier for me to live with the decisions. My parents' health had been an issue for years, with each of them needing multiple hospital stays. My mother had experienced several mini-strokes and the issue of dementia had been insidiously creeping into her life. We all knew it was a matter of time before my dad, with health issues of his own, would be unable to care for his wife.

Journal Entry: November 16, 2001

Well, that was a fast two weeks—or the longest two weeks? Anyway, much has happened. As expected, I got through it with God's grace. Report cards went home on time, and I just finished parent conferences. Always a joy.

I visited my mom and dad at the hospital last Sunday. There have been so many hospital visits over the years; this one seemed to blend together with the others. Then on Monday I asked my dad if Mom remembered my visit. "Tell me the truth," I said.

No, she hadn't was the answer. *That* is a harsh reality.

Today she was transferred to a nursing home. My brother called tonight to fill me in on some details. Since this was actually the third time in my mother's elderly history that she had been admitted to a nursing home, some of the process had lost its "wonder." On another occasion I had been the one to ride with her in the transferring ambulance, and my memory still stings with the freshness of that awful experience.

Since my brother lives so close to our parents, he, almost by definition, has to be the one to be there when most of this drama unfolds. So it was that John related how he had settled Mom into her new "home." And so it was that, as usual, I wasn't particularly surprised when the "zinger" came. I truly believe he doesn't do it intentionally; but so often something is said that makes me feel more guilt. Of course the problem may be I *am* guilty, so feel bad with good reason.

He was saying he wasn't sure what they'd do about Thanksgiving this year. I suggested they do it with his grown children as usual, since sadly my mother won't know the difference. He told me he was going to see about having it at the home. Ah. So, what am *I* doing? (He didn't ask.) As planned weeks ago, I'm doing Thanksgiving at my house this year. My husband's mother and sisters will join us.

Forgive me for going on with my life. I don't even know anymore where the line should be drawn. My life? My parents' lives? Ah well, I sense that I am just in a bad mood. It's been a hellish week. I *know* my brother had a rough week too, and although I've already promised to try to visit in two weeks (at his request so he and his wife can get away), he probably wishes I were there *now*. I cannot blame him for that.

I'm in touch enough with my own psychology that I realize all this bitchin' of mine is masking the issue I do not want to face: I am losing my mother. In most senses I've already lost her. Even our occasional phone conversations are discouraging. Yet she's my mother, and right now she's alone in a bed at some "home."

I don't want to think that she does understand what's going on. And I can't bear to realize that she doesn't.

Some pretty selfish thoughts really, but then they are *my* thoughts and feelings. I'm not always proud of them. I'm just glad God forgives me for them. And it was He who made me human.

Seven years my senior, John's always been the big brother, with all the implied responsibilities that carries. His proximity to our parents' house and his genuine concern put him in control of many issues regarding their care. Before my mother was admitted to the home, he and I talked about that decision, and I fully supported his conclusion that it was indeed time for her to be admitted.

On lesser issues (like should we hire a housekeeper), we would sometimes disagree on how to handle them. Certainly in the context of what we were now going through with my mother's condition, the feelings played out as usual. It was the needs, the relentless needs of those later years that wore us all down. Thank God, my brother and I were always able to put aside the skirmishes and misunderstandings. Maybe it was sharing the pain of seeing the parents we love go through what they went through that enabled us to focus on pulling together, not falling apart.

Journal Entry: November 29, 2001

So, my mom is in a home, and I plan to visit her there this weekend. I don't really expect this to be a cheery experience, but I am praying it will more positive than I think.

I hope to get my dad's Christmas stuff out and hopefully see that my mom is being well taken care of. Of course there is still the sadness of my parents' being separated, especially at Christmas time. I'm going to need some support and grace even as I pray for them and what they are going through. I will trust God to soften the hurt for everyone.

Christmas at our family's small house was always a festive time. My mother would hang these tacky plastic poinsettias up at the windows and deck the halls. A beautiful ceramic nativity set that her sister had made would adorn the hutch, and Mom would tape the Christmas cards up along the doorframes. Through the years the tree got smaller and decorations more sparse.

There were many years when my holiday memories were tarnished with illness and hospital visits. My mom particularly was sick a lot; my dad had his share of problems as well. Too well I remember eating Christmas dinners from a tray at the hospital. Once my mom pulled out the electric candles I'd put up when she and my brother were visiting my dad in the hospital. While I was only trying to persevere with the idea of Christmas joy, her reaction was understandable. Despite the inherent joy of Christmas, circumstances sometimes impose themselves, making our efforts to maintain that joy difficult.

Journal Entry: December 16, 2001

It's mid-December, the third week of Advent, and Christmas is around the corner. It was an okay visit to my parents' home in Rhode Island—actually, most of it was in Massachusetts, as I visited my mother in the nursing home in Fall River.

It's a pretty nice place—I guess, as those places go. She has a pleasant room with a large window and muted tones of rose-colored walls and draperies. Like I said, pleasant. Another gauge I use for judging nursing homes—and this is now the third my mom's been in—is the smell and the moaning. Both seemed minimal, so I was relieved.

We chatted some and took a slow walking-tour of her surroundings. Having my small camera with me, I took a picture of her leaning on her walker while my dad grinned his usual handsome smile. They *both* smiled, seemingly satisfied that this latest chapter in their lives was just one more bump in the road. (This photo appears in the photographs section.)

I held my mother's hand, and when it was time for me to leave, she told me she'd miss me. Yet I imagine she forgot I was there before I even cleared the Braga Bridge in Fall River, MA as I headed for home. Bizarre.

Now I expect to visit again next Sunday with my husband Tom. Our two grown kids, Michael living in New Hampshire and Jen who lives in New York, will be joining us. We'll do our "usual" holiday visit. Except it will be *un*usual, very different of course. I expect my mom will still be in the home, although permanent decisions haven't been made yet. Fortunately, the family can take her out for periods of time, so we will probably all go to a restaurant. Taking her to her house would likely be too painful . . .

My mother loved her little house. She would often tell the story of how she had saved up money when my dad was away in WWII. They'd bought this crummy little house that they expected to fix up just good enough to sell or rent out. Their real plan was to build a new one on the extra land that came with the house.

Then, as things happened, they found they loved the changes they had made and decided to keep the house for themselves. The land was divided and a lot sold off to my godmother. My brother and I were to receive the remaining two lots, but when it was time for him to build, zoning laws had changed and he needed my lot. I gladly sold it to him—I had no plan to live there anyway. Ah, the seeds of my ensuing guilt?

Journal Entry: December 31, 2001

My last conversation with my dad Saturday night was less than uplifting. Despite the fact that I had visited them just a week before, I somehow felt it wasn't enough. He'd had a rough day, has a cold, and my mother wanted to go home.

When we visited last Sunday, we did all meet at a restaurant. After dinner, we reassembled back at the nursing home, taking over a portion of an unused dining room. There we exchanged gifts, having to be content with the institutional Christmas decorations spread over the place. It was okay.

Being at my parents' house earlier didn't seem as strange as I'd thought it might be, maybe because I'd been there already without my mom being there. At any rate, I feel badly for my dad. My mom is in many ways already "gone"— which is very sad.

I find myself occasionally thinking this simple statement: My mother doesn't remember me . . . It makes me think of that "philosophical" question: if a tree falls in a forest and there's no one there to hear it, does it make a sound?

Of course, I remind myself, I don't *know* that she doesn't remember me. She just doesn't remember visits right after they occur. That's frightening really.

I think, as I pray sometimes, that if it's all the same to God, I don't want that to ever happen to me. We don't really know if she has Alzheimer's and I don't know if it really matters. But as for genetics (which I tend to downplay anyway), I'll tell you right now, *forget it.* I just smiled . . .

But seriously, if someday I'm in a home, and my kids ever read these ramblings of mine, pay attention to this:

"I will *never* forget you. My kids will *always* be loved by me. I may forget what you told me on the phone about your weekend plans, but *you* are too much a part of me that I will ever forget who and what you are to me.

Also, while I'm on this morbid subject, don't ever forget how much I love Christmas. No matter who's dead or whatever, always celebrate Christmas—string up extra lights for me, okay?"

Good Lord, I think I need to take a walk . . .

Dealing with death is one thing, but dealing with dementia is worse. At least I think so. Death is a certainty, and those of us with faith have the promise of paradise. Dementia on the other hand is this nasty game of chance. What is remembered? What is forgotten? Is it lost or just irretrievable? If I "have my mother's eyes" do I also have this illness lying dormant, waiting to claim me as another victim? Time to reclaim that faith I spoke of and take each day as it comes . . .

Journal Entry: January 4, 2002

I'm thinking I may go to RI this weekend–always an uplifting experience. Though now my dad is telling me not to come–so I don't catch his cold and "Besides, your mother will forget anyway." Thanks, Dad; I needed that. Yeah, that's pretty sad.

(Sigh) . . . Sometimes I think I need God to slap me upside the head. I have so much to be thankful for. It amazes me that He can forgive my bitchin' and at the same time provide some very needed comfort.

Journal Entry: January 10, 2002

Speaking of providing comfort—thank God for good friends! I met with my friend Kathy and unloaded a ton of feelings on her. Besides being a beautiful Christian and an old friend, she's a counselor, so I took advantage of "all of the above."

I confided to her that I thought I'd probably been repressing some heavy, sad feelings about my mother. Duh, ya think? She immediately zeroed in on some problems I was creating for myself—for example, by using terms like "I know I shouldn't feel this way," etc. She said, "Feelings are facts. They are just there, neither right nor wrong."

Also, in response to my lamenting that I sometimes just get the thought: "My mother is forgetting me," I should reframe that to say, "My mother's illness is preventing her from remembering many things, but she'll never truly forget *me*."

Additionally, she reminded me that my mother's condition is temporary. That as Christians we know life continues on the other side, and that then she'll be her old self again, and eventually we'll be reunited.

Thank God for such a dear friend! Of course I had some tears to shed. Even that Kathy supported as quite normal. The special circumstances of this stage of my mother's transition have put me in kind of a "pre-grieving" mode. Plus I *am* grieving the loss of my mother as she used to be.

Add to this some guilt that I've been praying she would die (because I don't want to see her like this) and some nifty fear that I could end up like her—well, it's a wonder I'm functioning at all. Of course some heavy-duty repression, denial, and compensation by humor have provided enough defense mechanisms that explain how I have. Not to mention the grace of God!

So, I guess I'll have to deal more with these feelings. Some crying has already helped. I'm planning to go visit my parents this weekend. My dad told me tonight he wants my mom to come home, so it should be an interesting visit. I haven't talked to my brother, but I'm sure I will. I'd better do some talking to God first!

Among the many pushes and pulls in the decision to place a parent in a nursing home is of course the other dear parent. My mother was eighty-eight when she was admitted to the home, my dad her junior by a year and a half. They were in their late twenties when they married, and we used to joke with them about Dad being younger.

Except for WWII, they were never apart for long. In their later years, the frequent hospital stays only made them more determined to stay together. When one visited the other during a hospital confinement, the visits would be daily and hours in duration. When this nursing home arrangement was thrust upon them, my father was still driving and went every day to see my mom.

Surely one of the saddest circumstances was when she would beg him to take her home. I'd witnessed this myself, and it would tear your heart out. I know for myself the visits were an

*emotional roller-coaster ride, with the plunge down always just
a little lower than it had been the time before.*

Journal Entry: January 12, 2002

I have to thank the Lord for what was actually a very nice visit with my parents today. I ended up coming and going in one day because snow was in the forecast for the next day. My mother, had she been herself, would have been the first to endorse this plan. She never liked me traveling if there was even a hint of bad weather.

Today I went to the house first and put my parents' nativity set away, which was a little sad. Coincidentally I'd put mine away this morning before I left my house. "Putting away Christmas" is always a bit of a downer, but knowing my mom hadn't even seen hers up this year gave it an added "ouch."

My brother came over and filled me in on several issues: Medicaid, our dad's car, etc. We all talked about Dad's wish for Mom to come home, and gently reminded him how severe her memory loss is, and how difficult it would be to care for her. Dad hung his head, and I knew that resignation was hard for him to accept.

Putting the heavy subjects on hold, my brother left to enjoy his well-earned reprieve from keeping his eye on Dad. So, my dad and I went to the diner at Kmart for lunch as usual— he loves their liver and onions. We actually had a good talk.

I found myself echoing to him some of the sound

judgment my friend Kathy had shared with me. He is understandably a little depressed about the present situation, but doesn't seem to be completely down about it all. I tried to be empathetic and offered some "reframing" suggestions that Kathy had advised me of. I also added the classic: "Try to see the cup as half full, not half empty."

Later, when my dad and I got to the nursing home, I was told my mother was in the dining room. At first I didn't see her in the crowd; then she saw me. I just said, "Hi"–didn't add "Mom"–just to test things. She immediately smiled and said, "Hi, Dear! I thought for a while you weren't coming, but here you are. I thought I may be dreaming, but when I heard your voice, I knew it was my darling Teresa." I offered up a silent "Thank you, Lord" on the spot.

There were several sweet moments like that. One of my favorites happened later as she rested on the bed. She made a general comment such as: "Oh, life is tough."

To which I, playing Pollyanna, said, "Well, it could be worse."

She then responded, "It won't be. I won't allow it." Somehow that struck me as a promise. Those things I may fear *won't* happen, and she'll continue to remember me.

As if all that weren't encouraging enough, she and my dad were especially sweet together–holding hands, kissing, singing old songs. It reminded me of last summer when they were in the car together going out for ice cream. Of course, much of this was bittersweet, and I fought back tears many times.

On the way home, I did cry some–not unusual and

actually I welcomed the opportunity. I willed myself *not* to think she'd already forgotten my visit. Instead I came up with an interesting outlook on it.

She is actually *not* forgetting things like today's visit—she's just burying them deep inside her. That's why she mentioned at first she'd thought she was dreaming I was there. She replays all the beautiful family moments in her sleep. It's like they're put in a safely locked box so she can carry them to the other side. Maybe she can't pull them out now, but that doesn't mean they're not there.

I suppose I'm recording this sweet and sad day so I'll have it to revisit, as I might need to in the days ahead.

Days like the one just described were true treasures. They became the hopeful promise that encouraged me as I approached each new visit. I never really knew how many more such days there would be, so I was thankful for them as they came. Even as I knew it would be difficult to see my mom in this environment and deal with her dementia, I tried to focus on the possibility of those sweet moments. The perseverance of their marriage was something I marveled at each time I saw my parents together.

Journal Entry: February 4, 2002

I got to speak to my mother tonight. She was all "How are you, Sweetheart?" although the conversation left a bit to be desired—like coherence. But this has been the case for quite a while. I ended the conversation with an "I love you," to which she responded, "I love you more." She even made reference to how she says that to my dad and they get silly with it. This is true, and I was glad she had the mental clarity to choose that response.

So, am I still awash in confusion and concern about my mom—and my dad as well? You betcha. At Mass yesterday I tried once more to really let it go—to God of course. I'm afraid I've been less than the victorious King's kid, and more the trampled down peasant. Poor exercise of my faith. I'm sorry about this, and I know God has not and will not exit this situation. And I know I must act on this truth.

It is distressing, but God is still God. That I have little or no control over what's happening to my parents at this stage of their lives just makes my surrender to the Lord that much more easy—and necessary.

To conclude—a quote I saw on a church sign: "No God, no peace. Know God, know peace."

Certainly one of the greatest gifts my parents gave me was faith in God. My mother particularly was a model of prayer and faith. Although I'd rebelled a bit in my college years, my own encounter with parenthood had brought me humbly back into the fold. I knew that despite any circumstance, God was in control, and that "peace that passes all understanding" would see us all through any crisis. It was just that my darn human nature would usurp these efforts of faith: "Lord, I believe. Help my unbelief."

Journal Entry: February 18, 2002

I visited my mom in the nursing home again today. And I've decided (at age fifty-two) that I *never* want to live in a "home." It sucks. I don't care how clean it is; I don't care if the staff is nice. It just sucks, and I never want to live in one. Point in fact, I don't think I want to live long enough to consider one. I'll hope God takes me out before then—please.

We prayed together, the three of us (plus God of course). I'd thought we might. I thought I'd try to do something positive, be some kind of cheerleader, shining light, whatever. So I suggested we pray. I stopped just short of asking aloud that God would take them home already; but surely He got my drift.

Mostly I thanked Him for a rich and wonderful life: the love, the faith, His care, and all that stuff. Then I made a point of reminding us that God hadn't changed, and although maybe now we were seeing the underside of the "embroidery that is our life," perhaps God would once again let us see the beauty and peace of it—from His point of view.

But as lovely as that prayer may have been, I soon heard my dad lament to my mom, "We *had* a happy life." Earlier she had said she wanted to die. Not exactly words on which to build hope and so forth. So much for the shining light.

It sucks, and I'm sorry. I told my dad—and I believe it—"Things could be worse." and "Try to take one day at a time." But truly, it is a very difficult experience.

The second day of my two-day visit had its "okay" moments. I spent most of it with my dad, even having lunch with him at the Senior Center. Then when I did go to see my mom by myself, I sadly realized I could have just gone on home, and no one would have known. But of course, I did go to the nursing home.

It was a nice surprise that there was a Mass at two o'clock, right there in the dining room. Prior to that I'd held my mother's hand and we "talked" a little about the good old days. Then I had to leave. I hugged her and told her I loved her. This was nothing different from any visit I'd had with her, except now I was leaving her alone in this place that isn't her home.

Then the dear woman says to me, "I'm sorry."

I said, "What are you sorry about?"

She says, "I'm sorry you're leaving." Then she starts to cry a little, and so do I. Then I stiff-upper-lip it and go . . . I try to expunge from my memory my mother lying on her bed with a soiled shirt, finding simple tasks of toileting and cleaning up difficult. Despite this being a good facility, the staff cannot catch everything. As a result, when I saw that spot on her shirt, I found it degrading, and one of the things I'd thought her being in a home would solve. Very simply, it makes me sad. But I am not the real issue. My mother is—and my dad. Their day-to-day existence matters more than how I'm "handling it."

Now I sigh "Paciencia" (pas-yan-sa)—the Portuguese word for patience. My God, this is very hard. *I'm* sorry, but it is.

One of the things that haunts my family is depression. My dad is bi-polar, and that alone makes for some grim realities. In her later years, my mother also experienced some depression, not uncommon in the elderly. With this backdrop though, it became increasingly important to me to recognize, express, and even justify my emotions. I'd learned already that denying them was a mistake, and fearing them perhaps an even bigger mistake. Better to explore and express these natural feelings and emotions and allow myself to be human.

Journal Entry: March 16, 2002

I'm thinking I need—somehow—to express the mixed emotions I have about my mother. Even as I try to relax on a weekend away at my husband's family cottage in Mystic, I am thinking: should I be visiting my parents? I do intend to—soon—I just hate to, that's all. All the negativity there impacts my motivation to visit. I am trying to make some sense out of it all, so maybe it will help to actually list how I feel about losing my mother and how my dad is trying to cope. So . . .

The guilt: Not being there. Asking God to take her—how can I wish my mother were dead? That's a major conflict for sure! Not being able to soothe my dad's grief. Seeing her in a place where, even though the staff is caring, she's not always being kept clean, safe from falls, or really "loved"—not as her family would anyway.

The sadness: I miss her—no more do we talk three times a week on the phone. I'm no longer able to really talk with her, letting her in on my cares and life events. Knowing it's downhill from here. Seeing my dad so down. There's loss—yet she is still here. A real tough one.

The fear: That she'll forget me. What that might mean.

That I'll end up like her someday—a stranger to my own family. I think I'd rather die first.

Should I "quit my bitchin'" and suppress? Or is that a problem for me already? Ah, the sweet mystery that is me. It is obvious that I have been wrestling with my parents' situation for several months. It is also quite obvious that I have a normal, natural avoidance thing happening—one that's really been building over the years.

Simply stated, I don't like visiting there—stuff, sad stuff, is in my face, and I'd rather keep away. I can only hope that's normal; who wouldn't feel that way?

So, all these feelings are just that: feelings—emotions, reactions, normal, allowed, and okay. Now I need to explore reaction vs. response and allow response to also be okay. I need to accept that my responses may not always be stellar—I mean that perfect, faith-filled, conqueror, up-on-top response.

If I'm down, I'm down, and it's pretty obvious that there's plenty to be down about. *Fortunately,* I also know I possess the ways and means to move through this experience. As usual I remind myself that other people suffer through much worse. And I do have so much to lift my spirits. I thank God so much for that reality and His truth that sets me free.

When people surpass the "life expectancy" figures, there are bound to be ambivalent feelings. How wonderful to still have your parents around! How much longer can they possibly live? When does quality of life kick into the equation? And how do we ever reconcile these questions?

Journal Entry: March 23, 2002

Well, heaven help me, I'll be off to Rhode Island this morning. I got a discouraging email from my brother yesterday. Mom is not doing well. She's losing weight and was sent off to the local hospital, but not to stay. They took x-rays that showed a fractured rib from a fall. But she also has a stomach sonogram scheduled for next Tuesday since there was a "blur" on the x-ray.

God forgive me, but one question that arose in me was "why?"–Why all the tests? Then later when I spoke with my sister-in-law, she said my mother may have had a heart attack, and my brother wanted to contact Mom's old cardiologist. Good grief!

We agreed my mother may (at last) be failing or shutting down–so why try to stop or prolong that? All this, along with some reports that my mother has uncharacteristically been using foul language lately, is pretty disturbing news. It should make for an interesting day.

Later that same day:

It was a rather extraordinary visit. As I drove there, I reflected on things and wondered if I'd end up talking to my mom. I believe we are entering the "final stages" of this universal yet distressing transition period. How we handle this is the variation, as everyone is different and circumstances vary of course.

As the visit began, it went well enough. My dad and I did his usual liver and onions lunch at the Kmart diner, along with a quick shopping trip for jeans for him. Later he and I enjoyed watching a basketball game on TV. In between all these activities, he talked a lot about my mom, how he wants her back home—to enjoy the new windows he got, their sunny deck, etc.

But then of course came the most significant part of the visit—seeing my mother. She immediately greeted me by name—yay! Things were going okay—that is to say I was doing all the talking. She was having back pain, so wasn't really up to walking or even sitting up much.

I rubbed her back; we prayed the rosary. My dad was there too, and I was beginning to think my mom and I wouldn't have any serious exchange at all. Then, toward the end of the afternoon, a nurse came in to ask me if my brother had found out the name of my mother's cardiologist. She began telling me how my mom was not well, and I signaled to her that I'd like to talk to her out in the hall.

There ensued quite a litany of problems my mother was experiencing: high blood pressure, urinary infection, and so on. Then she hit me with a whammy by telling me that if my mom continued to lose weight and not eat, then they'd be forced to suggest a food tube. And that this would have to be our decision.

I let her know how I felt my mother might be "simply" closing down, that at eighty-eight, she might just be getting ready to go. Although the nurse pointed out that they had people there over a hundred years old, she thought I was probably right. Still, they were obliged to check it out, thus the tests and so forth.

We talked at length—both in generalities and specifics

of how things can spin out of control. I asked her if she knew if my mother actually had a diagnosis of Alzheimer's. Going to my mother's file, she showed me a list of problems, with dementia listed, but not Alzheimer's specifically. Still, "a rose by any other name . . ."

The nurse had inferred my brother might want the food tube used. She also pointed out there was no legal paperwork beyond his okaying trips to the hospital. With my dad easily overwhelmed, it wasn't really clear who would be making these decisions should they arise. Then I did a wild thing.

I talked to my *mother* about it. My dad was dozing in the parlor, and I helped my mom back to her room where she could lie down. Then I just came out with it.

"Mom, you're eighty-eight years old, and you've lived a wonderful life. You seem tired, and I know you're not well. I'm wondering if you're thinking it's time for you to go to heaven to be with the Lord."

She said, "Yes, I think I am ready to leave."

I told her that as much as I would miss her, I would be ready to let her go. I wouldn't want to see her miserable. (She said she wasn't yet.) Then I even told her about the food tube and asked how she'd feel about that. She said no one had mentioned it, but she'd be "happy and proud." (??) I clarified by saying, "Well, would you want a food tube to keep you alive, or would you want to go on and be with the Lord?"

To that loaded question, she wisely replied that she wanted to be ready to go to the Lord when He says it's time. I joked that He might want to keep her here until she's one-hundred-ten. I asked if she'd been asking to live "just a little longer" the way she'd told me she used to do. She smiled as I teased that if she was holding out until one of my "kids" had a baby, she may have to hang around for a long time.

Then I asked her seriously if she was worried about Dad. She said, "No, I know he's all right. He's a good guy." I agreed and added that I believed that whoever went first would soon be joined by the other.

And then I said good-bye. I mean *really*.

I thanked her for being a good mother; told her that her most precious gift to me was her faith and how I hoped some day my kids could tell *me* that. I held her hand and prayed. I wouldn't have been surprised if she had passed away right then. Finally, I left her with my dad, saying good-bye to both.

Before I left the home I told that nurse the gist of our conversation. She was very supportive, saying she thinks I'd read my mother just right. I hope so. I mean at one level it saddens me to think she's failing, packing it in. However, my dad isn't on the same page on that at all.

I heard him say to her—and this broke my heart—"Don't worry, kid. I won't let you down. I'll have you home by the end of May." Then he added, "Even if I have to have a lawyer in here to do it."

Now I feel bad that he feels he has to take care of her, and I do wonder what his rights are as her husband. (Never mind that he's eighty-six and has health problems of his own.) I had asked the nurse about her possibly going home and us letting the chips fall as they may. She rattled off a list of dangers that would involve and that my mom really needed twenty-four hour care.

Sooo . . . Can I be sure she's failing because it's her time to fail—period—or are her surroundings the impetus? And if she could return to her little house, would it matter? Her overall sense of awareness seems mighty low. *Would* it matter? Even if it did, for how long would it matter?

It was an extraordinary day. Even though it was a distressing visit, I felt it was a gift. I got to say good-bye to my mother. Whether she dies in five days, five months, or five years, we already have some good closure. I have to thank God for that. And hold on for whatever comes next.

Maybe it's a generational thing, or a cultural influence, but our decision to put my mother in a nursing home was counter to our "gut" feelings and wishes. For most people it is that heart-wrenching decision that imposes itself, leaving no other real choice. In my mother's case, the "straw that broke the camel's back" was her toileting needs. The memory loss was a grave concern as she'd forget my dad had just gone out and climb stairs looking for him. But when she lost bowel control, we all knew it was over.

"Decision time" hit me between the eyes as I remember too well one day that I visited my parents at their house. My timing couldn't have been worse. Mom had just tried to use the bathroom and there was a mess. My dad made an effort to assure me he'd cleaned up everything and it was all under control. Then I saw the feces stuck in her sneaker, more on her foot. My heart clenched even as I filled a basin to wash her feet. There was no control. It was over. It was time . . .

So yes, she was admitted to a nursing home after that fall in November of 2001. But now, a few months later, here was my dad wanting to take her back to their house. What was best? What was even real anymore? And, darn that hope that sucks you back in just as you think you've resigned yourself to a situation.

Journal Entry: March 28, 2002

I'm getting sick of this journal reading like a bad melodrama. Get over it already! Yet, on the other hand, this may become a precious resource on this significant "passage" of my life. It wasn't intended to be a "theme" journal—I guess the theme would be "The Pain of Letting Go of Your Parents"—but it seems to be that.

Tonight I talked to my dad on the phone, and he immediately told me he's decided to get a lawyer and get my mom home. He saw her today and that's all she kept saying—she wants to go home. (I didn't ask if he was clear on *which* home she might be referring to!)

He continued with some off-the-wall comparisons of not putting a baby in a home because they mess their pants. To which I said there's a big difference in cleaning up a baby and a grown woman. Since other family members had been discouraging him, he took my comments as just more of everyone else's argument to keep her in the nursing home.

I did tell him I don't think he needs a lawyer to get her out—he *is* her husband. But if he wants to take her home in May, he needs to do the homework and do it right. He needs to figure out who and what they'd need at the house, because there is *no way* he could do it alone.

Then maybe he *should* take her home and let her die there. It's like what's the worse that could happen? I mean really, is she going to wander outside at two o'clock in the morning? More to the point, is she even going to remember her surroundings?

Can we allow my father to have this hope that she will come home—and can we even consider it seriously? I think we owe them that much. I don't know if I'm making any sense on this—I'm not going to be living next door and getting all the grief that would undoubtedly accompany her being back at home.

So, I put my dad off a little with the "in May" line (which he'd used before), and I'm thinking maybe she will go **home** (with a capital H for heaven) before we have to truly deal with that insane, impossible decision.

Journal Entry: March 31, 2002

Thank the Lord for a great birthday weekend, including today, Easter Sunday, here at the cottage in Mystic, CT. After my kids left this afternoon I tried to take a nap, but I couldn't seem to unwind. Key to this was the "flip side"—the unrelenting issues with my parents.

To cut to the bottom line, after a phone call with my brother, it's decided that Tom and I are leaving from here tomorrow to get me to a 10:30 AM meeting at my mother's nursing home. This of course involves calling in for a substitute teacher and having poor lesson plans. But I have to let that go.

Journal Entry: April 1, 2002

I'm a little wiped out and ready for bed. It was quite a day, but God was with me, and I am thankful for that.

The meeting was horrible—and yet it wasn't. My dad was loud and at times belligerent. I'm sure he felt outnumbered. He is also obviously "out of it." The head nurse finally told him how my mom won't be getting better and won't ever be able to go home. Ouch. I'm not even sure he was listening, although at the end he said, "Okay, I surrender. She'll be here till she dies." I tried to tell him that the news could be freeing for him—he *can't* take her home; it *isn't* his fault; he's a good husband, etc. Again, I don't know if he really heard me.

Then, when I saw my mom after the meeting, it was obvious they had been talking about getting her out. For the first time she told **me** she wanted to go home—maybe Monday (which was today). It was *sad*. I tried—gently, but uselessly—to remind her she couldn't have Dad take care of things.

What a sad state of affairs. It must be very hard for my dad to listen to that, and of course hard for my mother to feel hopeless. It made me think his surrender at the meeting may be quite short-lived. We'll see.

For such a long time my parents had really been taking care of each other. Now feeling that he'd let his loved one down, my dad was caught up in that real and painful reality of having his wife in a nursing home. So it is, that like any loss, having a spouse (or a parent!) away in a home requires the grieving process. And, as such, those pesky stages—denial, negotiating, anger—all come into play. Acceptance is a tease—flitting in and out, until something triggers the cycle again.

Journal Entry: April 11, 2002

The visit with my parents this past Sunday and Monday was as hard as I'd thought it would be. I logged six hours at the nursing home the first day. Mind-numbing to say the least.

After lunch on Monday, I went to the nursing home by myself, bringing my mother some cooler clothes. As visits go, it was okay. I do not feel the need to repeat my good-byes (from March 23rd). In fact, it seems odd she hasn't left yet.

I know I have to deal with this strange grieving process, but for now I think I'm "okay." Since the meeting on April 1st, and my dad's "acceptance," things seem to have settled somewhat. Of course that can change at any time. I do want to thank God for the visit though, and for reminding me that my parents are His children.

Journal Entry: April 21, 2002

I didn't sleep well last night, but at one awakening, I revisited an idea. This "ending" of my mother's life is somehow a kinder transition for those people who love her. I'd actually been thinking of my daughter Jennifer and how throughout her life I've had to let her go. I remember—vividly—the various stages of that process, particularly her college years. It was hard to let go, and surviving all that with her made it no easier when I had to repeat the process with my second child, Michael. Still, I can recall telling friends that God was good and merciful in that the process of letting your children go was a gradual one.

I saw, once again, that letting my mother go was also a critical transition. With death often being unpredictable, we don't always have a transition period. Now my mother is definitely transitioning her way out of this life. Over the last few years, and most definitely over the last few months, she has been slipping gradually but certainly *away*.

Already I have lost most of what was our relationship. Phone conversations, encouragement, advice, jokes, shared concerns—long gone. Oddly, just now I remembered labor pains when I had Jen. She took her time coming. Then when labor truly began, she was born within a few hours.

As my mom is exiting, it's like that somehow—drawn out.

Journal Entry: May 2, 2002

I'm writing now in hopes it will help dispel the stress I'm feeling. The thing is, my dad called tonight. He said he had some sad news—my mother fell—again. Poor guy had gone to the home yesterday and found my mother on a stretcher. They were taking her to the hospital for x-rays—nothing was broken.

Good grief. How miserable for both of them. Now she's barely getting up to walk, he said. How much more are they going to have to go through? I'm sorry, but I think I had managed to put some distance between the day-to-day reality and myself. (It's called self-preservation.) It comes crashing in again, and I'm incredibly sad. I just can't stand to think of my mother (and Dad too for that matter) going through the fear and pain, loneliness, and so on and so on.

So, whether good, bad, healthy or not, I've lately tried the "denial" phase, tried to "back-burner" the whole situation. But it just doesn't go away. Why am I failing to let this go truly to God? Why haven't I reached that "peace that passes all understanding?" I know God is comfort. Please let Him comfort *them* first—then me.

Journal Entry: May 12, 2002

It's Mother's Day, and I saw my mother this afternoon. As visits go, she seemed a little "better" than last time. Still, conversation just doesn't happen. My dad left almost right away to go back to the house, but he and I had a good chat later . . . I suspect this may be the last Mother's Day with my mother, on this side of heaven anyway. I'm asking the Blessed Mother to welcome her with open arms—soon.

Journal Entry: May 13, 2002

My brother had told me yesterday that Dad, who is diabetic, had experienced a "near-miss" with his blood sugar dropping very low. My dad and I talked some this morning, and he told me that his "near-miss" felt kind of good—just like falling asleep. We agreed that sounded like the way to go. I don't mean we were being morbid or suicidal; I just mean he sounded reflective. I told him some about my "good-bye" talk to Mom back in March. He even got a kick about my teasing her if she was waiting and living to see Jen or Mike have a baby. He also acknowledged that Mom is getting weaker.

When we arrived at the home today, my mother was asleep. He woke her up with a kiss, and right away asked her who he was. She answered, "You're my darling husband." He smiled and gave me a "See that?" grin. I was less courageous, but said something to her like, "Okay, now I'm the tough question." To which she said, "You know who I am." This of course, didn't make sense, but that's about how things go. Two hours later I kissed them both good-bye—and had my cry.

Losses were in abundance in these months of my mother's

passing. Well beyond the physical loss of her now living in a nursing home, there were the emotional losses raged by her dementia. Simple contacts were eroding, and she was slipping further away. Memories of silly phone conversations or more serious mother-daughter sharings were bittersweet. Maybe we tend to follow the words of that song, "The Way We Were"— remembering the laughter, the good times. Maybe that tendency is just good mental health—substituting better times for the ones now holding us in darkness.

Journal Entry: June 5, 2002

My mother has entered yet another phase, I think. My dad says she can barely walk, so they brought her wheelchair to the home. I haven't seen her since Mother's Day, and frankly am hoping to put off a visit till after school is out. I *think* I'm numb, and then something simple sets me off in tears. Case in point:

Last Monday I was in for a medical exam. I wore my gray sweatshirt—my mother had embroidered little flowers around the neckline. When the nurse asked if I had done it, I simply said, "No, my mom did." Then my eyes filled with tears. My mother didn't even know I was there. She didn't pray for me, as she always would do. (Or did she?)

What world is she in? I still can't stand to think about what level of consciousness she's in right now. I just can't.

Journal entry: June 17, 2002

Tonight I got to talk to my mom. It was so nice to hear her voice. It had been a long time. I miss her. Really. Even though I know she wasn't really processing my comments, it's like I needed to tell her about my day like I used to. She sounded good, in good spirits too. Then I talked to my brother . . .

He told me she's scheduled for a colonoscopy in July because there was a shadow or possible mass shown on an x-ray of her hip. Could this be her ticket out of here? I hate to even think of her going through the prep, and of course I don't want her to "go out" in pain.

So when did God last consult with me on how He should run things? I know, I know. He must shake His head at my fretting. I know too that I have managed to "back-burner" my parents' situation lately (just to get through the day-to-day school stuff). Now I know it will come crashing down around me. I do know He'll see me through it though. He always does.

Journal Entry: June 23, 2002

I must thank God for a really good visit with my parents today. In fact, I just wrote an eight hundred-word personal essay on it on my new laptop, which Tom convinced me to get, and persuaded me to take along to RI today.

I don't want that to take the place of this journal since I do like communing prayerfully with God. Still, I am finding the writing is providing a welcome release from feelings.

~~~~~~~~~~~~~~~~~~~~~~~~~~~~

The "Endless" Ending

Although I continued to write in my prayer journal regularly, including of course my concerns and conflicts about my mom, I began to use my laptop, taking it with me each time I went to visit my parents. Then, after my dad had gone to bed, I would sit up in my old bed upstairs and literally pour my heart out. Usually within an hour or two I'd be left with a personal essay I could revisit if I chose. Though sometimes different in tone from my prayer journal writing, each one was still my immediate reflection on what had transpired. Some essays I shared during a writing workshop I participated in from time to time; others remained totally private. Regardless of the format, the essays *and* the journal entries simply told the recurring story of the sorrow and sweetness of seeing my parents during these visits.

Now, for the remainder of this book, I present my essays as a chronological account of the remaining time my mother lingered in this life. I am painfully aware that they record but a tiny portion of what her experience truly was. I know also, again by definition, that these personal essays reflect my perspective, flawed as that might be. I cannot apologize for any of that.

Instead I suggest that they might inspire reflection as to how much of life we do let go of *without* recording it or reflecting on it. If writing saves things, as I believe, then not writing might seem to lose things—and not just things, but life itself. So, in the following pages, I offer up some fragments of what were my mother's last months on this earth—at least the way her daughter saw them.

Personal Essays

Families dealing with dementia know that the path spiraling downward isn't a predictable one. Even in the course of an hour or certainly in a day, the person stricken with dementia can vary in degree of confusion and distance. Sometimes you get a "gift," only to have it snatched away. The teasing of time and experience leaves you hoping for more. This first essay reflects that frustration and hope.

What If She Forgets?
Essay: June 23, 2002

Every time now, when I go to visit my mom in the home, I sort of hold my breath when I first see her. It isn't that I'm afraid of what I'll see, although there is some of that. Since I may see her every three or four weeks, the time that has passed *is* an issue. But what it is, what I'm really afraid of, is that she won't remember me.

I hold my breath, half expecting a "Who the hell are you?" Thankfully, that has never happened–yet. So today, when that moment comes, and she responds to my "Hello" with a "Hi, Dear," I take it gratefully.

Now I'm not stupid. I know that as brave as I was to leave off the "Mom" on my greeting, her greeting was rather generic as well. So another moment passes, and it's as if I'm playing "chicken" with myself. How close to that cliff do I want to go? At what point do I bail and say, "How are you, *Mother?*" before she does come out with a "So who the hell *are* you?"

But this day I'm batting a thousand. There's a nurse or aide or somebody in the room, and my mother turns to her and says, "This is my daughter, Teresa." And my heart beats again, and now it's soaring. I smile, for I've been gifted one more time. I am thankful, praising God in the silent recesses of my heart.

This day, this time, my mother remembers me again. I can tuck the nightmare away once more. I can believe, as I want to so desperately, that she's not getting worse, that she will beat the dementia that is robbing her blind of the most precious part of her life: her memories.

Let her forget when she had her hair done, as she tells me later she has. Let her forget how long she's been there. God, let her forget countless bits of her personal history, but for the love of all that matters, let her remember me.

This time she does, and I am profoundly grateful.

Later I receive a bonus. During this visit she is actually having some fun, teasing a little. My dad is sitting dutifully by her bedside holding her hand when he launches into a sweetly dramatic recital of how and why he visits her every single day.

"I don't want her to forget who I am," he says. "When I come she seems happy to see me and she remembers me, so I keep coming. Right, dear?" he adds, looking up at her.

She stares back blankly.

"Who am I?" he asks her, and I find myself holding my breath once again. "Do you know who I am?" he persists.

"You're a pain in the ass." She says deadpan, then grins. We all burst out laughing.

Later still my dad leaves the room to check on her nightly medications. He worries about this because sometimes if he tries to leave before the meds are given, she won't let him go. She'll beg to go home, and this naturally breaks his heart. The medication seems to soothe things over, and he can slip out quietly. But they're understaffed this Sunday evening; the usual nurse isn't there. So Dad goes out to check.

"Where'd your father go?" my mom asks. She asks this as soon as he leaves, even though he's just explained where he's going. I wonder if I'm in for it now, and we'll play the "who's on first" game of confusion.

"He went to find a nurse, Ma," I explain patiently. "To see about your pills."

It's her turn, but she says nothing, just screwing up her face. Her face, which now resembles a crumpled brown paper bag, gives no other clue as to where this conversation is going. So I go ahead and take another turn.

"You have a doting husband." I tell her.

"Dopey?"

"Not *dopey*, doting!"

The crumpled paper bag is crinkling and shaking

slightly. She's laughing at me and her wonderful joke. I laugh too, delighted that she's having fun with me.

Finally a nurse is found, and pills are given. A kiss all around and my dad and I are ready to leave. When I ask her if she minds us leaving now, she answers with some twisted explanation of why she has to stay there anyway. I think there's some reference to a door prize that she has to be there to claim. Sadly, I realize she's lost again, the bewilderment bubbling to the surface once more.

"See you tomorrow," I tell her.

"Okay, Dear."

I leave with a smile on my face. It's been a gift of a day, a really good visit. And I will see her tomorrow.

I wonder if she'll remember me.

A month later and I'm off again to visit. There have been updates via frequent phone calls with my father of course, as well as talks with my brother. The phone calls where I talk to my mother are few and far between. Always underlying the decision to visit is the guilt, which has been a plague for years. Always ready for self-examination, I try to meet it head-on. Yet I know guilt isn't the real issue; it's loss and it's grieving. And it's unrelenting when a parent slips so slowly and sadly away.

Seeing My Parents
Essay: July 17, 2002

I'm going to see my parents tomorrow. That's probably why I can't sleep, why I feel like plodding down to the kitchen to eat a few hundred crackers with peanut butter, why I feel a little lost and a lot sad.

I can't recall exactly when visiting my parents went from a happy thing to something equivalent to having a root canal. But then I've never had a root canal, so maybe that's not an honest comparison. I just know the visits lost the fun, became a burden and an obligation, and finally a painful thing to dread.

Naturally one cannot have those feelings without mixing in a good dose of guilt. How *can* you feel that way about visiting your parents? I just do, so I guess I can.

There was a time when as a grownup person, married with children, it was a trip back in time to bring the family to the old homestead. To allow the parents to "ooh and ah" over the kids, to plan the special meals, the visits to the cousin's pool, the long and lazy chats in the backyard under the willow trees. To watch your children run through a lawn sprinkler just as you had a million years before—that is a connection and an emotional trip worth taking.

But time changes things. The parents got older, which is sort of strange because I, of course, did not. It seemed as I returned home I was stuck in time, ever the good daughter, seeing reruns of life's little dramas unfold before my eyes. I could still talk about my hopes and dreams and all the silly unimportant events in my life. My parents always seemed to care about all of it. As much as I derived attention from these visits, I know my parents enjoyed them as well. It worked for a while, but in time not so much.

How does all this get to be about me, I wonder? It's their story, their decline that precipitated the lost joy, the feeling of "Oh no, I don't want to go there." It started of course with more frequent trips to the hospital, a sad throwback to my teen years. I have a collection of orange plastic basins that represent a fraction of my mother's hospital stays. (She could keep the plastic tubs and things, and of course these weren't ever thrown away—someone could use them.)

So the pile of basins added up, and the visits were less than joyful. Over time my parents grew ill, and somehow in my selfish twisted head it was all about me. I would have to go there and experience those feelings that I just didn't want to feel—the dread, the powerlessness, the fear, the loss. I hated hospitals and I hated visiting them.

Fortunately, a couple of decades later, there was a reprieve. Maybe it was the awful state of affairs in hospital care, maybe it was improved health, maybe it was a small miracle, but the hospital stays leveled off. Now it was back to the home front, where I could see my parents shuffle through their rooms, painfully climb the porch stairs, and even more frightening, drive off to McDonald's every morning for coffee and a bran muffin.

In time, my own children grown and moved away, my travels back in time were made alone. My husband opted early to stay at home, and this really made more sense. I didn't need to add the tension of his boredom to an already uncomfortable event.

So, I'm an awful daughter, who never looks forward to visiting her aging and ailing parents. I remind myself that there have in fact been good visits, but realistically I know that's only true because I've lowered my expectations so much. There have been a few pearls among the stones, but the rarity of that occurrence is less than encouraging.

I sigh and think of all that has gone before. There were good times; there can still be precious moments. With my mom now in a nursing home, and my dad struggling to come to grips with everything that entails, it seems maybe it's a good time for me to get my head together and think more of them for a change. But maybe that is exactly my problem.

I *do* think of them and what they are each going through. I think of the past, and the present seems a bit too intense. Raised to have faith in God, I see us all forgetting to involve Him in the nitty-gritty of what this transitional phase has become, the daily fears and foibles that mark their lives. The invitation to pray is one I still bring up, but there's a strain there, one that seems to have only recently developed. It has something to do with the need for that "peace that passes all understanding," when understanding is lacking in spades.

I still don't want to go tomorrow. It's been nearly a month though, and of course I really need to go. My dad will be glad to see me. We'll go to Kmart (yes, Kmart) for lunch, as this has somehow become a ritual. We'll go see my mom and sit there for hours until I can almost feel my brain atrophy. With any luck, she'll still remember us and hopefully won't cry to come home. That would constitute a good visit.

I've learned to lower my expectations. But what kind of attitude is that?

Maybe I need to readjust my vision, see things not as they once were, not even as they are now, but somehow, with the eyes of faith see beyond to what they will one day be. This is a transitional time. I am sadly and completely human in my selfish sadness and emotional desert. Only God can make it right. Only the promise of paradise can make this present holding pattern bearable.

I need to remember my expectations are dictated by the events of this world only if I allow them to be. I need of course to pray, and in praying draw comfort, a comfort that will sustain me and hopefully spread to the people who need it even more—my parents.

I hope it will be a good visit.

When compiling these essays, I couldn't help but notice a big gap in time between this last essay and the one that follows. It needs to be noted that while all this was going on with my mother, there were other difficult life experiences happening as well. My son went through a painful divorce. My Dad's depression reared its ugly head and he was hospitalized. He and I visited, but I didn't write about seeing my mother.

In my prayer journal I referred to this time as the "3-D Effect"—a Dying mother, a Depressed father, and a Divorcing son. The continued journaling captured my emotions as life provided faith and fear their chance to dominate these circumstances. I did find an August journal entry that recorded some reflections on my parents. I'll include that here and then return to the essays; for my mother's story pressed on, and I continued to visit of course.

Journal Entry: August 1, 2002

I guess I should record some thoughts and feelings I experienced today about my mom. I was watching a brief segment on a TV news show and the subject was Alzheimer's. A woman's daughter began to say how she missed her mom who has the disease and how her mom used to hug her. I immediately started to cry. I mean it sort of amazed me how right "out there" that emotion was. It was total empathy and total recognition of my ongoing grieving.

Then tonight on the phone my dad was sweet as he related how my mother was cuddling with him on the couch today. They haven't been able to go to the parlor there as much, and I'm just now realizing how that must be yet another loss for them.

Mom is still losing weight I guess. They gave her a smaller wheelchair since she was practically falling out of the other one. Dad told me she cracks her eye open a sliver when she's dozing on the bed to see if he's still there. He once said how sad it is that "She'll be there forever." I do pray for him—that he may be comforted.

Visiting Again
Essay: September 28, 2002

Here I am again, sitting up in the bed I occupied as a kid, at the old homestead. As usual I dreaded coming, and as usual I was blessed with a moment. Seeing my elderly parents holding hands, hanging onto life together, and playing their game of "I love you—I love you more."

She greeted him warmly, reaching out both her hands. He took the too thin fingers into his large hands, and as she said, "My darling husband," he said, "My darling wife."

I just sat there as if caught up in some corny movie, somehow an intruder in this tender moment, but one who couldn't turn away. I knew it was yet another gift, a moment to remember and to treasure, and maybe even to envy. How many people can claim that much love sustained over that expanse of time?

No, I didn't want to come. I'd had a hellish week myself, and the need to take care of myself seems to be more real to me as I grow older. Still, we all are pressed into facing the realities of life. I knew I had to come and would make it through okay.

Earlier, my brother and I had discussed the sadness surrounding our parents' lives now, and that maybe living past eighty-five for them just didn't seem worthwhile. We discussed how "medical science" has loused up the human race. Were people living too long? How can anyone know the answer to that?

Certainly as a family we all do what we can, and no one is suggesting "pulling the plug." It's just the mystery of this prolonged passing that has us stymied. We talked about how they aren't in pain, yet even tonight my father said, probably for the millionth time, "Who knew it would end like this?"

Indeed, who knew? And when will it truly end? Indeed, who knows?

Surely a significant part of my mother's last years of life was her new environment. As with many of the elderly, especially those no longer able to be cared for at home, she was in a nursing home. Her surroundings, as well as the people there with her, played a role in every drama to unfold during each visit. I saw this world as an outsider. A world of both hope and despair. It was a world I'd only travel to, with strongly mixed emotions, my stomach always in knots, a false smile planted on my face. Each time I wondered what I'd encounter, both with my mother and with those other poor souls.

The Last Visit?
Essay: November 9, 2002

It seems that every visit with my parents over the last five years has potentially been the last visit. Today's was no exception, with this reality thrown in: it must be getting damn close, that last visit. There can't be many more.

On entering the nursing home, I asked the nurse where my mother was. I was told that she was in the dining room, so I joked that I'd try to pick her out among all the other white-haired ladies who looked pretty much the same. But I saw my mother quickly, saw her head down on the table, and knew I had stumbled in on one of her tired times, where all she wanted to do was put that head down.

I went over to my mother.

"Wake up," I said, "You've got company."

She looked up, smiled, and said, "Hi, my darling." Before I had a chance to judge whether that was purely a generic greeting, a man who was visiting at her table remarked, "Oh, she was just talking about you."

That sort of threw me. "Really?" I said. He responded by saying she'd told him I visit every now and then. Later I was to wonder if I should have questioned him further. Had she been truly talking about her daughter or just responding generally to a question of his? This can seem important as I agonize over what level of awareness she has. But I let it go.

My mom was glad to see me and glad to see her husband. It was sweet to see her fuss over him, asking for a kiss, then a bigger one and a bigger one. I almost wondered if she was showing off a little bit to the other old ladies who don't have husbands any longer, but that I'll never know either.

We talked in that around and around way I'm getting used to. For my own selfish reasons I shared some news, just wanting a reaction from my mother. She did pretty well, especially when I told her my husband Tom and I are planning to buy his family's cottage in Mystic and move there. "You do it," she said. "Grab it up!" She had always encouraged me to hope for Mystic some day, and I knew her feelings were genuine.

But I don't kid myself. She won't remember the

conversation, probably won't remember that I was even there. But at least for that moment I was talking to my mother and sharing dreams with her like I used to do.

At one point my mom and dad had both nodded off to sleep as I sat at the table playing Bingo with the room full of geriatric cast-offs. That's rather harsh, I know. Many did seem totally lost and one lady in particular got my attention. She rolled herself right up to our table and began pleading something in Portuguese. I tried to explain I couldn't understand what she wanted. I tried to get her past us, thinking she just wanted to get through the tangle of wheelchairs, but that wasn't it.

Finally her gestures made it clear. She wanted my hand, and when I gave it to her she drew it to her lips and kissed it, a sweet smile on her face. I hugged her—then did so again. Meanwhile my dad was awake now and started complaining that she was a pain in the neck, and I needed to roll her over to the other side of the room.

This I did, though not without some sadness. I told my dad she was a "pitiful pain" and indeed she seemed to sum up the many personalities in that large room. Once again a visit to a nursing home had created for me a travel experience on which I would rather not embark.

As I've noted before, this place was probably better than some others. Efforts were made to keep the patients occupied, with the staff available to help. Visitors were always coming and going. But the people, the old people, they seem to be waiting for something that never comes. Whether you think it's a visit from a family member or a call from God Himself to come on home now, it's a wait that you can sense and be pulled into before you know what hit you.

My mom today was among those waiting. She cried a little when I first arrived. Ever the coward, I ran off to use the bathroom, and sure enough, when I returned she was under control. Several times during the visit she said, almost in a singsong voice, "I want to go home to see my mother and my father." They have of course been long dead.

Even when I gently reminded her of this, she continued to tell me, "I want to go home." I thought what I've thought before: she is ready to go to heaven. "You pray to God, Mother," I advised her, and I told her I would too.

Is that sick? Is that cruel? Or is that just the reality of having a nearly ninety-year-old mother whose quality of life is so reduced she can't remember who visited her today and never thinks to ask about her grandchildren. She is waiting, along with all the others. God's waiting room, they call it. When will God say, "Mary, your turn to see the Great Physician; come on in."

I hope she won't have to wait much longer.

One of the things family members grapple with as their loved one struggles on with dementia is when will it end? Unlike a specific disease ravaging the body, this evil grip on the brain seems to take its time, teasing with windows of hope and slammed doors of discouragement. Add to this the guilt of longing for an end to the anguish, and you've got a formula for some pretty trying times. It's not unusual either for family members to differ in their feelings as these circumstances ultimately result in "decision time."

It seemed to me my brother often looked through rose-colored glasses. For him there was always one more thing to try, one more procedure to sign on for, even as I wondered what were we signing on for and for whom? These differences sometimes tempted the two of us to yield to the growing tension and argue. Most often though we both admitted our basic uncertainty, and tried to exercise a faith in God's timing. This itself can be an arguable point: when do we stand in the way of God's timing, prolonging death, not preserving life? Yet, if not for an underlying faith, how can anyone face such decisions?

My Mother is Dying
Essay: January 1, 2003

I've been thinking recently of death. I know that sounds morbid, but I don't mean it to be. With the sad but inevitable progression my mom has been taking, I've just been wondering more about that transition from life to death.

When does living become dying? I mean, at what point in the human experience does a person stop living and start dying? I'm sure there are medical road marks that define the process more precisely, but for the layperson, the average person, what marks the change over? Whatever it is, it seems my mother is now embarking upon this final leg of her long journey.

Surely after all these months of failing health and

rapidly diminishing mental capacity, she hasn't truly been *living* for quite some time. Now, with the relentless weight loss, has come dehydration, and everyone knows a person can't live without water. In whatever stage of reasonableness, the nursing home asked about inserting an IV, and my brother, bless his heart, said okay to that.

Within a half-hour my mother had pulled it out, and we, her family, were left looking at each other, knowing she had made her choice. And we must respect that. It is time for her to depart this world and finally, thankfully, pass on to that place we believe in as Christians—heaven—where there is no more pain or tears or suffering. It is time to let her go to be released into that white-light tunnel that leads to peace and the presence of God.

I saw my mother three days ago, and I knew then she'd pulled out the IV. She was sitting, as she often has been these last months, with her head down on the table, hardly aware of her surroundings. I had come to visit for the holidays, this time with only my husband with me as the children had gone back to their homes. A virus being present at the home had thwarted an earlier visit with everyone else. (With my daughter now pregnant, we were unwilling to risk her getting sick.)

So it was that I sat by my mother now, feigning happiness and teasing her to sit up and enjoy her company. I gave her the Christmas packages, and she did a good job expressing surprise and delight in her gifts—two pairs of sweat pants and a small teddy bear angel. Then came the good news—the news I'd probably anticipated telling her for a very long time.

Despite the fact that my brother had already told her

about my daughter, I'd joked that I would still have the happy privilege of telling my mother for the first time. This was basically true, so I told my mother that my daughter was pregnant.

She clapped her frail hands and said, "Oh goodie!" A nice reaction to be sure, but to be accurate, I should add that she first asked if the news was that Jen was getting married. I had to explain that she had been married for three years. My mom and dad had even gone to the wedding. But background stuff is lost, and I knew even this exciting news would be lost as well–probably in the time it took for me to say good-bye and leave my mother once again.

This leaves me on this New Year's Day with reflections on the past year: saying good-bye to my mother more times than I can count. Even now I consider how gracious God has been to let her live through the holidays, thereby not scarring Christmas even more than it has been in my past. How selfish is that? Pretty selfish, but since I have prayed to God about taking her *now*, I know I was being selfish last week in asking that He *not* take her then. Since I've long realized God doesn't listen to me on that prayer anyway, I figured I had nothing to lose in asking for a week's reprieve.

So today, when my brother called with the update, I should not have been surprised by what he told me. In fact, there was little real change in my mother's condition, but what had changed was our reaction to it. At the home, she is now on "Comfort Care." No more IV, no more blood tests, just keep her comfortable. There was a meeting the day after I was there and decisions were made toward that end. Hospice will step in and meet with the family, the home will provide as dignified an experience in her death as they can.

My brother assured me he would keep me updated, having no real knowledge of when my mother will die. I remind myself that she and I said our good-byes last spring. I remind myself that I have cried and felt despair with her condition for months. All this is so much past history as I face the present circumstance.

My mother is dying.

My tears are there as always. I can tell myself it is a blessing, and it is. I can remind myself of how rich and full her life was and how dear our relationship was. I can even praise God that I had the chance to tell her that my daughter will be having a baby this coming summer. I can do all those things, but I will still cry for the loss of my mother.

There is something quite profound I think in the circle of life that is being completed. As my mother prepares to die, my grandchild prepares to be born. That is quite miraculous. Being in the stage of life that I am, I see the cycle clearly. It's the yin and the yang, the sad news, the good news, the dying and the being born.

For everything there is a season. My mother is dying. My daughter is pregnant. There is loss and there is gain. There is joy and there is pain. I know I will miss my mom, but I also believe she may feel closer to me when she is in heaven than she has seemed in recent months. For that I can be grateful. So—

"Good-bye, Mother. I hope you will see your new great-grandchild from your spot in heaven. I suspect I will be asking you for some advice from time to time. I will miss you, but I have missed you for over a year now. I hope I can be a good grandmother, and I thank you once again for your presence in my life. Enough. Good-bye already."

An area I touched on after my last essay was some occasional disagreements between my brother and me. Certainly caring for elderly parents can be an emotional minefield for relationships. There is no doubt that my brother is their primary caretaker. Being a virtual back-yard-neighbor to my parents has won him that dubious honor. The years where that proximity benefited him most have long gone. Instead, he is the one to get the phone calls in the night, the one to fill the pillboxes. Now, with our mother in the home, he continues to look after our dad.

With two grown children of my own living a significant distance away, I try to balance visiting with them with my obligations to my parents. Often I plan my visits specifically to relieve my brother if he requests a certain time frame. For the most part he and I seem to relate amicably to this geographically dictated distinction in our roles. He has admitted he's limited his own visits to the home, finding them depressing, of course. So I guess we both struggle with some guilt in maybe not visiting "enough"—however that's even defined. But I'm the distant one, the absent one, and this fact feeds my guilt relentlessly.

Guilty As Charged
Essay: January 19, 2003

It's been nearly three weeks since we all got the word that my mom was dying. And she hasn't died—yet. With conversations with my brother about coffin linings and refreshments after the funeral, it seemed all that was left was laying aside the right clothes and all would be over and settled— and life could go on.

Well, maybe not so much.

What *has* gone on is the sadness and tension and terrible guilt as I consider what to do and when and where to do it. My mom hasn't died, and I am, as always, extremely conflicted as I debate with myself: Should I visit? Can I avoid it? How bad a daughter/sister am I anyway?

Perhaps it's time to look more deeply at what leads me to this emotional abyss. I don't know who originally wrote this refrain, but it could be my mantra:

You can, you can't;
You will, you won't.
You're damned if you do, and
You're damned if you don't.

To be immersed in guilt and indecision is increasingly becoming my modus operandi. I suspect it stems from the plain fact that I *could* be doing more toward taking care of my parents. That my brother pretty much has that covered only enhances the guilt, since he obviously does so much more than I do. It's impossible for me to ever catch up.

So, is this just sibling rivalry? No, I think not. If it were,

I could make a good case for my contribution by trying to step up what I do. Maybe I could visit more. I suppose I *could*, but I don't really *want* to. Oh, there are several really good, logical reasons why I can't visit more often, but they seem to look rather self-centered when taken in the light of what's going on over there.

Admitting I don't want to go seems pretty upfront to me, and I haven't been struck dead by a lightning bolt for not sufficiently "honoring my mother and my father." Maybe I can poke at that reasoning a little.

I don't want to go there.

Who would? Generally it's an unhappy place where unhappy things are happening. As a grownup, I am expected to toughen up and do what I have to do. And, in my defense I do that, averaging once a month visits to the homestead. I drive the nearly two-hour trip, battling Providence traffic and crossing some emotional time zones to arrive at the house I grew up in.

The house is minus my mother and is haunted by my dad who wanders through the small rooms alone. My brother's house is literally a stone's throw away, and many a visit has been outlined by his report on "the situation as it stands." I see the dirty bathrooms and the drapes hanging sloppily and I wonder how my dad manages at all.

Then, just to add more emotional depth to the visit, I drive to the nursing home where my mother has been living–or dying, depending on your point of view–for over a year. I've pretty much gotten over the fearful expectation of her remembering me or not. She seems to, at least marginally. (Although last fall when I called her on her birthday and she told me "I forgot your name" —well, that was a real kick in the heart.)

It is the certainty that she will forget I was ever there within minutes of my parting that unsettles me. I, on the other hand, will remember in horrific detail every sight and sound and smell of the visit. In fact, it is without success that I try to expunge from my mind some of the memories of my mother that each visit provides.

I don't like to go there, but I do go there. And sometimes I don't. I have a choice. Seems to me this might explain the conflict, might explain the guilt, might even explain the relentless pondering of what I should do. What should I do?

There's the now famous question: What would Jesus do? Well, I suspect He'd visit more regularly than I do, maybe even cross Narragansett Bay without benefit of a bridge. In truth, I try to pray about all this, ask Him for help, for strength, for wisdom. It comes, but in dribs and drabs and filtered sadly through my wretched humanness. What would Jesus do?

Perhaps a better question to consider as I wrestle with the guilt is: What would my mother do? Or perhaps, what would she say? When I allow myself to really think about this, I come to the conclusion she would let me off the hook. Despite wanting me to visit of course, she was always one to worry about my safety and my needs. If there was a snowflake in the forecast, forget it. A rainy day? Don't come! She'd often suggest a phone call instead of that long ride alone. I can't ask my mom though, as she is sadly past conversation.

Yeah, my mom would let me off the hook. Sometimes I call my godmother to get her opinion, or more honestly to have her back me up as I verbalize my reluctance to spend another weekend visiting my aging and ailing parents. So I put it off a little longer, still averaging that once a month visit, knowing full well whenever I do go it will be depressing as hell.

My brother lives right there. He has no choice. I do. I feel guilty; he likely feels resentful. What a lovely arrangement. I'm beginning to think that guilt, like sadness or anger, is just one more emotion we have to live with. At times it can drive us to change our behavior, but mostly it just sits on our heart and ebbs through our brain, doing nothing but spoiling the pleasures of the moment. Like sadness and anger, self-destructive but unavoidable.

What does it matter really? All this emotional garbage and debate, and I am no closer to understanding what it all means or why it all matters. Feelings, a friend once reminded me, are neither right nor wrong, they just *are*. I want someone to tell me I shouldn't feel guilty, but maybe I should. I know I *do*, so that is probably all I need to deal with right now.

I am guilty as charged.

Déjà-vu All Over Again
Essay: February 20, 2003

I approached the nursing home with some trepidation. After all, it had been nearly two months since my last visit, with not even a phone call with Mom in between. Oh, I had all kinds of reasons why it had been so long—everything from snowstorms to flu bugs, but that was hardly the point. What mattered was—would she remember me?

Since I'd been visiting my mother over the last fifteen months at this "nursing facility," I would often wonder if this visit would be the one where she'd look at me and say, "Who the hell are you?" In fact, an encounter last fall had dealt me a blow with her comment, "I forget your name." So okay, I had reason to worry.

Yet, despite this genuine concern, I had not been prompted to push myself to visit earlier. Perhaps somehow I knew one of two things would happen: she would either remember me or not. And either scenario seemed perfectly understandable, and therefore acceptable.

I am amazed, as I often am, by how God works things through. He tends to move extremely slowly, giving out bits of life that may indeed hurt, but can be tolerated in small doses. So this awful wretched good-bye with my mother, although a torturous process, seems to have hardened me to the hurt just by its duration alone.

But I digress.

I was visiting today, and I wondered if she would remember me. At first my dad, who was with me, decided to take a detour through the hallways, letting me go on ahead of him. This I did not like, since I felt having him with me would set up a natural context in which my mother could at least place me. I was fussing with the elevator buttons when my dad appeared anyway. That problem solved, we stepped off onto my mother's floor together and set about trying to find her.

She was in the dining room, her head resting on the

table as it always was. She looked up as my dad greeted her, and I, ever the coward, mumbled a, "Hello, Mother." as I kissed her forehead. She, in turn said, "Oh, my darling, I'm so glad you came."—just as she had many visits before.

Later I received a bonus when a Hospice volunteer came in to visit her. She went on and on to him about me—"This is my daughter. Her name is Teresa. She's a good girl. She's my only daughter . . ." It was reassuring I suppose that she did obviously remember me, and nothing had changed. She was no better, but no worse.

Despite alarms sounding several weeks ago—thus the Hospice involvement—my mother apparently has reached some sort of holding pattern. My fond and emotional farewells can all be repeated because she isn't dying, at least not now. That this does not particularly comfort me belies my heart—hurt or hard, I cannot say.

I just know that as I sat there through another three-hour visit, I felt caught in a time warp. It was last fall. No, last summer. No, last spring. I felt as trapped in time as my mother is. Instead of feeling grateful that I still had her, I felt the continuing sadness and loss I have felt for well over a year. I haven't had her truly in all that time.

So the visit was the same, the nurses the same, the news the same. Someday there will be the change, the one we wait for, and I know when it comes I will cry and maybe even long for these visits. But not today. Today I just feel the sad sameness that is this long good-bye.

Postscript 2/22/03

I visited my mom the next day as I usually do. The second visit seems to be the one that rattles me, probably because from there I leave for home. And when I say good-bye, I don't know when I will see her again. When I arrived this time, she greeted me as the day before, seemingly glad to see me.

Not long into our non-conversation, she told she had cried that morning. She said it matter-of-factly like some people might share they had seen an old friend.

"I cried this morning," she told me.

"Oh?" I responded.

"I do that sometimes. I cry and cry. I cried, but then I couldn't remember why I was crying."

At that her crinkled face twisted wryly and we both grinned. She made some comment about that making her feel worse, but it was obvious to me she saw the humor in it too.

I laughed and said, "So, you forgot why you were crying? Oh well." We both smiled at the bittersweet farce this all was. She was at that moment the mother I had always had, sensitive and funny, and ever the fighter.

I was grateful for that moment, and others that followed. I got to tell her yet again that my daughter was pregnant and she seemed to fixate on that for a while. Somehow it got twisted up in her head and she asked me to go get the baby. She asked me a dozen times if it was a boy or a girl and when it was due. Later I left a note for the Hospice nurse telling him the silver lining in having to tell my mother *again* about my daughter: I got to see her excitement over and over each time she got the "news."

So my mom and I talked, in pieces and in parts, in stops and starts. Sadly, thankfully, I think I am getting used to this dance that is talking to my mother.

Then I had to say good-bye of course. I said it as the entertainment that afternoon provided a backdrop of the song "You Are My Sunshine"—one of the songs my dad always sung to her. I knew I couldn't last through that, so I got up.

"I have to go, Mom. Bye."

"Oh, don't go," she said

"I need to go. Be good. I love you."

Her face twisted and she put her head down. I turned away before I could see if she was crying. I knew she'd forget I had even been there within twenty minutes. As usual, I cried as I left. I sucked it up in the elevator and let it out in the car. I cried as I crossed the Braga Bridge out of Fall River, but I made myself stop so I wouldn't get creamed in Providence traffic.

I cried most of the way home. And sadly enough, I could remember why.

A Different Visit
Essay: March 22, 2003

Visiting my mother in a home has been my unhappy practice for going on a year and a half now. Most of the time it seems I'm in some sort of time continuum where things are the same. I'm trapped along with her as we wrestle with some sad semblance of conversation or connection. But today was different.

She greeted me the same, with a "Hello, my darling," that leaves me strangely uncomfortable. In its wake I struggle to determine if she in fact recognizes me or is just smart enough to know this generic greeting will get her through the first minutes of our meeting. A month had passed since my last visit, with no phone calls anymore, no outside connection. I am always braced for a "And who is this?" from her lips. But again, today was different.

Within minutes of my arrival, she turned to the quiet woman beside her at the table and said, "This is my daughter, Teresa." (She first said my name in Portuguese, which she rarely does.) The woman, who had the sweetest, though most vacant smile I've ever seen, looked at me shyly, as I politely acknowledged this introduction.

Her name is Mary, as it seems to be for half the female patients at the home. She quickly tuned us out and reentered whatever world had her attention this day. I looked again at my mother and waited, waited for the next statement, the next interchange. I had decided I was not going to press this time. Let her reach out to me. In some twisted and probably unwise way, I needed to know the extent that my mother could still do this.

I will confess here, that a good part of my reluctance to open up and initiate an exchange with her is the price I paid last time. A month ago I had the pleasure of telling my mother *again* that my daughter is pregnant. On that day there was little else to say to her, so I rehashed it several times, and despite some disjointed questions on her part, she seemed genuinely excited and interested in the baby. With some Pollyanna attitude in place, I told myself later that this was really kind of nice. I had some fun telling my mother all over again about the baby, the ultrasound pictures, and the joyful preparations. That she seemed a little fixated on it didn't concern me at the time; it only underscored how excited she was. Or so I thought.

The following day I was back home, once again immersed in my own life, when I spoke with my father on the phone. He matter-of-factly told me my mother was okay, but she now thought she was having a baby. I was aghast. Ironically, months ago, a friend of mine at work had told the story of someone in *her* mother's nursing home who thought she had just had a baby and how sadly funny that was. My dad assured me it would pass and he wasn't worried about it.

I was not so much worried, as I was disappointed. So much for Pollyanna. What I had seen as a silver lining–the ability to tell and retell my mother this happy news of my expected grandchild–had somehow gotten twisted in her twisted mind so that she thought it was she who was pregnant. Not an easy feat at age eighty-nine. And yes, I joke here of course. It was a joke, though not funny at all, and a circumstance that caused me to have my visit today without mentioning the baby at all. And, of course, she didn't ask.

So, on this day, at this visit, I held back, waiting to see what she would have to say. When she did talk to me, I was struck by her words and alarmed at her candor. She told me she had been feeling depressed this morning because my father wasn't there and she had wondered if I was coming. In fact, it had been two days since my dad had been there, but she made it sound as if he had taken off just that morning without telling her where he was going. She slipped in and out of the reality of where she was, but it seemed painfully clear she was aware she was alone and was most certainly feeling lonely.

This pulled at my heart and placed a weight of dreadful disappointment over it.

When I am away from my mother, for reasons I know involve self-preservation and mental health, I like to believe she is only in the moment, not realizing how long someone has been away. She's not missing anyone. She's not feeling the desolation of being left in this place that is not her home. A place where she is being cared for by people who are not her family.

Today's visit was different. When I spoke with Mom's nurse later, telling her some of this, she remarked casually that my mother's medication was being readjusted, and she may indeed be more or less conscious of certain things. Really, what had made me think we could go our merry way thinking my mother is in "her happy place," in limbo, not lonely? What made me think this prolonged separation could be anything but incredibly sad and undeniably unkind?

Yes, I visited my mother again today, and the thing that was the same was that I learned something. Each visit seems to bring a lesson, usually unhappy or bittersweet. Today was no different. But I am forced to face the fact that this visit held a revelation that I would have chosen not to experience. My mom is lonely there and misses us and misses me and thinks of me, and maybe even pines for me. At least I know she pines for her husband.

Throughout this exchange today, my dad sat just a few feet away and blessedly retreated into his hearing loss (I hope!). He didn't seem to hear a lot of what my mother was saying. Later, when I tried to talk to him about it, he changed the subject rather quickly, but not before I managed to tell him how hard I know it must be for him to leave her.

When she is aware, she presses, wants him to stay, wants to go home. How he can stand it, I have no idea. My experience today was enough to set my heart back a few beats. I advised him, as I had before, to always kiss her good-bye (just in case). But now I acknowledged that if necessary, he should leave any way he could.

Still, today's visit wasn't all doom and gloom. I asked her if she wanted to pray with me. She quickly said yes, but added, "You do it. I forgot how."

I took her hand and prayed, thanked God aloud for what had been a nice visit today. Then I asked, as I always do, for His "peace that passes all understanding." I stopped short of asking Him to take her home—home to be with Him where she need never feel lonely nor neglected. I've pretty much given up trying to tell God what to do. He doesn't seem to need my advice on a myriad of things. So I wisely remind myself He's not likely to care too much about how I might suggest He run this situation.

Visiting a loved one in a nursing home is probably one of life's most painful experiences. "Parting is such sweet sorrow," and today was certainly no exception. I didn't want to sneak out like my father sometimes does, but after trying to explain things to her, I realized his way had its merits. Still, knowing it would be a few weeks before I saw her again, I didn't want to leave in a lie.

Finally, the best I could do was to persuade her that Dad and I had to get some dinner because we couldn't eat in the dining room with her. This is all true. Of course I didn't tell her that we wouldn't be coming right back. My dad had left already, and at last she seemed satisfied with my good-bye kiss and my "I love you—very much."

She echoed the same to me and put her head down on the table. I patted her head and hoped she wouldn't look up, wouldn't see me grab my jacket, wouldn't realize I was heading for the elevator, hadn't said, "See you later."

As I left her behind in the dining room, my heart was in my throat, tears prickling behind my eyes. As I pondered what had just transpired, I knew I was faced with two possible scenarios, neither one a comfort. I knew that she would either forget I had even been there, or she would be left wondering why I hadn't come right back. For her sake, I hope the former, and experience tells me this is the more likely reality. I ponder a lot.

If a tree falls in the forest and there is no one there to hear it, does it make a sound? If I visit my mother, and within minutes she's forgotten it, where in the time continuum does it exist? I guess it must reside in *my* memory, a responsibility I will gladly assume, especially if it lightens her load of loneliness a little.

And so, the likely scenario is that this visit is long forgotten, and she resides in the moment. It is the less painful scenario for her, I pray. It is also the scenario that leaves me now the one left most alone.

Yes, this was a different visit.

I suspect that the many little dramas I'd witness when visiting my mother were also playing out in any nursing home anywhere. I noted with wonder (and yes, guilt) a woman who seemed to always be there with her elderly mother. I learned they'd lived together and the daughter was committed to daily and extended visits. There were few men around, as patients or visitors. Wheelchairs lined the nurses' stations. Smells of disinfectant made futile attempts to hide urine—does aging flesh emit its own odor? On top of the angst I felt in seeing my own mother here, so contrary to what we had hoped for her final years, I had glimpses of the lives of other residents—too many too sad.

Again, Yet, Still
Essay: May 31, 2003

Riding up in the elevator together, my dad and I feebly joked about where we would find Mom. Of course, I hadn't been to the nursing home in a month; but he, ever faithful, still averaged three or four visits a week, so he had the advantage. (If you could call any deeper knowledge of what goes on there an advantage.) Still, he had told me she often wheels herself around in the wheelchair. He finds her usually by the nurses' station or maybe by the water fountain.

Our sad attempt at "Where's Waldo?" came to an

end soon after the elevator doors opened. There were lots of patients and visitors milling around, but no sign of my mother. I craned my neck around the corner and peered into the dining room where I spotted her at her usual table. Thankfully she wasn't resting her head on the table this time, but seemed to be interacting with a young man standing nearby.

As my dad and I walked in, we were greeted by the sad sounds of a nursing home, those haunting wails that ring throughout the air in every place like this on the planet.

"Hell - puh! Hell - puh mee! Pul - leese!"

It was the same woman I had heard almost every other time I'd come, and a part of me wanted to tell her to just shut up. My earlier reactions had been more sympathetic, but I had since learned that there wasn't anything really wrong with the lady. It wasn't like she was being neglected or anything. She was probably just putting to voice a deep need that no one—patient or nurse or visitor, really wanted to hear. Especially so loudly and so damned repeatedly.

"Hell - puh !" She stretched the word "help" out each time. I wanted to block my ears. It was no surprise when a few of the patients did tell her to shut up—in at least two languages. The wailing paused, at least briefly.

Meanwhile, I approached my mother. As usual her eyes went to my father first, and my heart ached a bit at the love and yearning caught up in her voice when she greeted him. She called him darling, in Portuguese, and demanded he kiss her again and again.

I had come around the other side of her, and when she turned and saw me she smiled broadly—or at least as broadly as one can smile when one has no teeth. I was safe, realizing she remembered me. Once again the dreadful fear that she would not know me could be put aside.

As visits go—and there have been so many I cannot count them—it was typical. Sad and funny and mind-numbing. My mom and dad were sweet together. She wanted ice cream, so off he went to get some. The three of us sat silently spooning too-soft strawberry ice cream from 4 oz. Styrofoam cups.

It felt good on my scratchy throat, yet all the while I was remembering towering ice cream cones on hot summer days when Dad would drive to the town creamery. They would go every day, just for an outing. Whenever I'd visit, I'd happily go along, seeing a corner of their lives that was as sticky-sweet as the ice cream dribbling down Dad's chin.

But that was a long time ago—no, just two years ago—before my mom's last fall at their house, before she began to lose control of her bathroom needs. It was before their lives took the twist, the turn, the unraveling that has brought us now to a small table in a large dining room, with Styrofoam ice cream in 4 oz. cups.

The ice cream eaten, it seemed my mom decided it was time to fold the paper napkins, and refold the cloth bib someone had left lying on the table. As I watched my mother persevere at this mindless activity, taking care to match corners, my dad looked at me knowingly. "She used to fold clothes in the shop," he said, referring to decades earlier when she did some factory work. I could see her at home folding dishtowels and sorting the laundry, even up to her last days there. Was she seeing herself there too?

Meanwhile, "back at the ranch"—there was no Bingo today. That disappointment alone seemed to echo through the room, as I heard several patients talk about it. "No Bingo." "It was cancelled." "Everyone's gone today." "Oh well." Several more heads bobbed down on chests. May as well go back to sleep. May as well check out for a little while longer. What was there to do anyway? No Bingo today.

Within our little threesome, our own drama was playing itself out as my father told my mom we would have to leave soon. "Oh no," she said, "The iron that was here has just sunk down to here." As she said this, she held her thin hand to her heart and dropped it to her stomach. I knew then that this was not to be an easy visit.

Despite some off-track comments and such, my mother was in high awareness mode today, and that meant leaving was going to be painful. Of course the leaving has always been painful, but when she is aware, she won't let you leave. You have to either lie or leave her in tears. I chose a compromise—a little white lie.

Sending my father out ahead of me, I told her I would check with the nurse about her medication. Then I walked blindly to the nurses' desk, tears already brimming my eyes, without an ounce of courage to look back.

"Damn, this is not getting any easier," I said to the head nurse. She and I talked briefly about the sad reality of this. My tears spilled over when I asked her to tell me the truth: "Does she remember sometimes? I mean after I leave."

"Sometimes," came the answer, and my heart broke with the truth and the horror of what I knew but didn't want to know. Too easy to believe my mom is just in the moment, and it is true, she mostly forgets right after you see her. I've seen evidence of this time and time again. Like today even—there was no, "So where have you been?" from her. No sense of time lapse. Getting easier? Not by a long shot.

And so, again, yet, still, I cry and I grieve. I tell myself that life is for the living, and I have to just go on and live my life. My mother was lost to me in most ways years ago. Yet today, as I held her hand, I wanted to will her back to us. Her smile, her fear, her loneliness were all there exposed to me, and I wanted to scream, "Hell - puh! Pul - leese!"

But someone probably would have told me to shut up.

Time of course offers perspective, and as I consider the following personal essays I wonder if God wasn't preparing me again for the final good-bye. In His wisdom, which to us ignorant souls can at times appear cruel, He lets us know that death is not the ultimate suffering. As my family had been dealing with the random meanness of dementia (Alzheimer's or whatever it was!), the recurring experience of loss was a torture.

A few years before, when my mother was first experiencing her memory loss, I'd asked her if when she "lost" a particular memory was it all truly gone or was she always struggling to retrieve it. She told me then that it was "just gone." I was comforted in knowing that, at least for her at that time, there wasn't the added suffering of feeling it lost and being powerless to get it back. The suffering then was experienced more by those people she loved, those people she'd seemingly forgotten.

September Mourn
Essay: September 6, 2003

It had been a good two months—quite literally a *good* two months—since I had seen my mother at the nursing home. Though not intentional, the length of my absence made sense, given the busy activities of the summer—and my grandbaby's birth had provided a great distraction! Also I *had* managed to see my dad when he visited us in Mystic. I just hadn't gone to his house, where I would have gone to see my mom too. In other words, I'd managed to tone down my guilt pretty well. Then came today.

It was time, and I knew it. I'd spent some stressful moments last night just in dreadful anticipation of what I knew lay ahead. I figured there were three possible scenarios to play out when I'd see my mother: 1) She wouldn't remember who I was; 2) She would remember and cry that I'd been away too long; or 3) She'd react indifferently, in the moment only.

None were particularly pleasant, but, feeling like I was in a bad game show, I was personally hoping for "door number three." Alas, the first scenario greeted me with only a touch of choice three to complicate things.

When I arrived, with my father close behind me (I figured the familiar backdrop of my dad would increase my chances of being recognized), my mom looked up from where she'd been resting her head and said to me, her only daughter, "Who are you? Are you my sister?" Ouch. When I responded "No," she said simply, "Oh, I thought you were my sister Agnes."

This would have been troubling enough if she *had* a sister named Agnes, but there too her sister *Sarah*, had she been with me, would have also suffered a disappointment. Anyway, seeing that I was not her "sister Agnes," she just resumed her favorite position, her head on the table, closing out all that was around her, including my dad and me. Ouch again.

In the fleeting moment when she had looked at me, I was stunned, not only by her misunderstanding of who I was, but also by how she looked. Beyond the emaciated, harshly crinkled old face, there was a new misery to behold. I'd been warned she'd been "picking" on herself, pecking at pimples or sores till they bled. Sure enough, there on the center of her forehead was an open sore. It was about a half inch wide and added to her already pathetic appearance. Later I noticed dried blood on her fingertips.

All things considered, I knew I had stumbled into my nightmare. This was not to be a stellar visit. In time I saw it had nowhere to go but up. And I have long ago learned to lower my expectations.

My dad sat beside her and pressed his luck a bit at my expense. "Don't you know Teresa?" he asked.

She picked up her head long enough to say, "I don't know anything about Teresa." The blow was painful and I wanted to run. But I sat rigidly in my chair.

Moments later when my dad left to use the bathroom, I set off once again to check reality—a sucker for punishment, I suppose. When I asked her flat out, "Who am I?" She said, "You're Thruhsa-bluhsa."

I smiled. That was the Portuguese nickname she'd had

for me. Later still she called me Teresa, and of course I was relieved. I put the earlier, painful comments aside, as I clung to what I had received. It was some note of recognition, some connection—though sadly fragile to be sure.

Determined to salvage more threads of this visit, I showed her the pictures I'd brought of my new granddaughter. Again, since my expectations were low, I was happy to hear her generic responses of "How cute." Long ago she had stopped asking about my grown children. But I knew her love for them was buried deep within the recesses of her aging, jumbled mind.

Perhaps that's not right. More likely the love resides within her heart, my mother's heart that was always full to overflowing with love for her family. It's locked inside her heart, though her brain is shorting out the signals that would allow her to express it in ways we have always treasured. In ways we've not seen for a very long time.

On this September morn I felt, once again, the mourning I have experienced for years now. Years that my mother has been lost to her family and me. Seeing her today was probably more painful than seeing her dead in a coffin. In a coffin she would not be suffering, and of course I would not be expecting her to greet me, recognizing me as her daughter.

Instead, I got to once again experience that long good-bye that tears at me, my father, my brother, and all those who love my mother. The good-bye lingers, as sadly we remember what she does not remember: the life she had and the way she truly was.

The woman I saw today is not my mother, not really. Yet of course she is. The conflict and confusion her condition creates are unrelenting. The emotional roller coaster each visit provides is a bad dream that seems to go on forever.

At one point today, my mother said, "I wish I would die." I tightened my jaw before I could say, "I wish you would die too." What sort of exchange would that be? What sort of feeling is that? But what sort of life is that? I do not know.

I only know I grow weary—as does she—of this endless ending to my mother's life.

Maybe This Time
Essay: November 1, 2003

This time, when I stepped off the elevator at the home, my dad just two paces behind me, the nurse at the desk looked up right away. Almost imperceptibly, she beckoned me to her, and said in a soft voice, "Did anyone call to tell you she's not doing so well?"

Considering my mother has been "dying" for at least ten months made the question just short of ludicrous, but I knew what she meant. "My dad told me when he visited on Thursday that she was in bed and getting oxygen." As I said this, I turned to look at my mother's bedroom, where the door was now closed. I was told they might be changing her or some such thing. The nurse began to look through my mother's file to give me the latest updates.

"Not doing so well" seemed to hit the nail on the head as I learned she has pneumonia with both lungs affected. She had been receiving antibiotics and oxygen for three days now. They'd had her up for a couple of hours this morning but now she was in bed. A part of me wanted to ask why they were bothering with the treatment, but I knew already that what they were doing was hardly extraordinary. It had to be done.

That my mother's departure from this earth was once more being delayed came as no surprise to me. That she was in bed was different, but I had braced myself for this. So I approached her room as soon as the door opened.

A wizened creature, raisin-faced and insanely thin, lay in the bed where my mother was supposed to be. I had been considering just this phenomenon as I drove the two hours to get here this morning. My mother, I'd decided, had been removed from me about two years ago. In her place was this pathetic stranger who, although her voice was remarkably still my mother's, when she spoke, her words were not. And her body was surely not.

My mother had been small, a short and chubby lady with wrinkled skin, but a ready smile. This person who lay in her bed seemed to sink into the mattress, though not with weight, but waste. Plastic tubing invaded her nostrils as a nearby machine hissed and bubbled in its noble task. Fresh oxygen supplied to a ninety-year-old woman who has been asking to die for the last two years.

I approached the bed.

Taking up the small hand, I said hello to my mother, knowing the mind game I was playing would not take me far. This was my mother, a fact I alternately avoided facing or hit head on, depending on my state of mind. Within moments I decided I needed to take a Xanex, a medicinal crutch I allow myself sparingly and almost exclusively in relation to my encounters with my mother. I decided this occasion warranted at least a quarter tablet. But I would wait awhile and allow myself to feel the rising anxiety and hopeless sorrow. This time it looked like my mother was really dying.

A "cat with nine lives," my mother has been so close to the brink, and so many times, that anyone in the family is always at a loss to feel loss—because she doesn't leave. But maybe this time. This time might be the last time I see her alive, the last time I get to hold her hand, the last time to tell her I love her, to listen and wonder and hope she'll have some last words for me as well.

She has words, as I lean in to listen, but they are mostly indecipherable. As the hours pass, I catch snippets of clarity, a "Praise the Lord" here, a "Thank you" there. At one point I wonder if she is asking to see a priest or oddly mumbling "my freezer." Is she telling me she's cold? Or—and this occurs to me much later—is she saying "my Teresa?" Another mumble, and I hear, "I can't live much longer." I search her face and try to assure her that's okay. Later, however, when I ask if she's getting ready to go to heaven, she clearly answers, "No."

This time, as in other times, I am not to be graced with words from my mother that I can cling to or remember with peace. She dozes and tosses. I hold her hand, thinking it's too warm and way too thin. I check with the nurses again and receive the now familiar shrug that means anything from "Have you contacted a funeral home?" (Yes, we did, ten months ago) to "Who knows; she's a stubborn old lady." (This too I know to be true.)

Throughout this visit, my father sits nearby, eyes focused on his wife's face. He complains that she isn't looking at us, seems fixed on the window on the other side of the room. I wonder what she's seeing. The classic "Walk toward the light!" comes to my mind as I watch my mother's eyes gazing beyond us.

I find a rosary by her bed, and decide it might be a good idea to pray it aloud. I do, by myself, wondering if she'd pass away right then and there. Later, when I think my mother might be asking for prayer, I sing some favorite spiritual songs, and she seems a bit more subdued. Again, I wait for the final breath. I can hear the rattling lungs so close beneath my hand as it rests on hers over her shriveled chest.

The fractional Xanex seems to have taken the edge off, so I sit fearlessly by my mother's bed. I hold her hand and try desperately to hear what she continues to say. But her voice is too soft and the words are so jumbled, only angels could decipher them. I hope I am not missing some last endearing incantation. I soon realize that is wishful thinking on my part.

Later, I encouraged my dad to sit where I had been sitting, where he could hold her hand and hopefully hear her if she chose to speak to him. I watched as the image of my father's huge hand gently covering the frail fingers my mother offered him imbedded itself into my memory. The tender gesture, as so many others, stood in testament to a marriage of sixty-three years. Was my dad thinking as I was, that this might be the last time he gets to hold her hand?

I never really expected to be with my mother when she

dies, since I live so far away. That my brother probably would be seems more likely, since he lives literally in their back yard. This week my brother is in Florida at a wedding, hoping to stay another week to enjoy some well-deserved rest.

Meanwhile my mother's turn-for-the-worse is still open for interpretation—will this go on for two days, two weeks, two months? I have no intention of calling my brother—I don't even have his number, as he left one of his grown sons in charge of communication. The nurse says she'll contact him and me if need arises. I'm not sure how that has been defined, but later when I prepare to leave, I tell her I'll be stopping by again tomorrow.

The last few visits have found me wanting to avoid the second day, but this time, this time I think it may well be the last. This time I want to bring my mother a scapular, that religious cloth sacramental that my mother (good Catholic that she is) "always" wore around her neck. I know she would quite literally "never be caught dead" without it. When I asked a nurse if she'd seen one, she thought for sure she had, but neither one of us could find it in her room. Now it seems important to me to get her one before she passes on without it. Though not personally devoted to Our Lady of Mount Carmel (and the graces promised to those wearing the brown scapular), I vow to search the house for one tonight.

But now it is time for us to leave.

My dad and I check in with the nurse first since my dad seems worried that my mom keeps pulling out the oxygen tube. She has done this several times since we've been there, so I check with the nurses on this point. They assure me it is not keeping her alive, so if she takes it out it won't make much difference. Open to interpretation? Still, I relate this to my dad, and he appears relieved.

The visit is over. Standing by the elevator I find myself leaning forward, trying to peer around the corner. I see my mom in her bed, thin hand near her face. She's fingering the oxygen tubes, wanting what? To pull them away, to take a final breath? To rest, as I told her to do, or to leave as she must?

The next day, I do return, this time without my dad. My mom seems worse, her skin clammy, her eyes barely opening. Again there's mumbling and I strain to hear her—no good, nothing I can understand. Although my search for her scapular had failed, once again I find her rosary. I pray it aloud and see her mouthing the words. A few times she even blesses herself, and I am amazed at this perseverance of prayer.

Perhaps too soon, I decide it's time for me to go. I feel as though I have given her a chance to pass on while I was there, but that wasn't to be. With the long drive ahead of me, I decide, as I know she would, that it is best I leave before dark.

Placing a kiss on her sweaty brow, I again say good-bye to my mother. Seeing the nurse, I remind her to call me, and she assures me she has my number. I am in the elevator when I remember one more thing. Almost embarrassed, I head back to the nurse's desk.

"Do you know," I ask her, "if my mom has had a priest in to see her? I think she might have months ago, but I'm not even sure."

"I'll check on that," she says kindly. "Don't worry."

Don't worry. To myself I admit I only worry that my

mother would want any spiritual send-off available. And I don't want anything to prevent her from leaving, especially leaving peacefully and "prepared." The endless ending that has become my mother's life may at last be fast approaching closure.

I drive home, sorrow enveloping me as it has so many times. Although surprisingly tearless, I wonder if maybe this time my sorrow will yield to mourning a real death. Maybe this time it will not be locked in the loss that has held my mother for these two years—not an actual loss of life, but the dreadful loss of living.

Maybe this time. I await the phone call.

The Phone Call
Essay: November 18, 2003

The phone call came this morning, just short of two weeks since my last visit with my mother. When the phone rang, just after 6:30, I had just sat down with my decaf coffee and whole-wheat bagel. Of course I knew it was the call I'd been waiting for.

My brother's voice, soft and familiar, was soon telling me what I already knew: our mom had died, just moments before. Gently, he told me some details: that he had been with her praying the rosary; so she wasn't alone when it happened. Within minutes we'd exchanged reactions and the barest of proposed plans. When we hung up, I saw the time was 6:38, and I set about doing what I had to do.

That I cried—hard and inconsolably—surprised me a little. Since my mom has been virtually dying for months, it struck me a bit strange that I immediately felt such sadness. I found myself relieved I was at home and not at work where I had said I could take the call if necessary. My husband Tom wasn't even with me, being away on business, so maybe that helped in a way to just free me to experience that moment myself. The moment you learn your mother has died.

Naturally, I had to call to arrange for a substitute teacher at work. Then I did call Tom; then my brother called back. In fact there were a few calls from John as plans for the day unfolded. He had thought he'd keep the news from Dad for awhile, but circumstances did not permit that. I'd already decided to head right over there, so I quickly got things together—really most had already been packed, so I was on the road before 9:00.

First I had to call my kids though. I tried Mike first, but there was no answer. Fortunately, I did reach Jen, and we talked about how they could possibly come to the funeral. The baby was sick, so that didn't help matters. I didn't want to lay any guilt on her, but I did suggest ways to do it, as we felt of course she should come.

Two hours later, I was holding my father's hand, trying to console him as he cried for his life partner, his wife of sixty-three years. I was glad to be there at my brother's house to connect to the family at this time.

My brother and I went to the funeral home after lunch to make arrangements. That experience was hardly an edifying one, but suffice it to say we got the details taken care of, and walked out with a bill for nearly eight thousand dollars.

Other "highlights" of the day included looking through my mother's things for her best rosary and underwear to go beneath her pink dress—all to be brought to the funeral home later. There were some light moments though, while in the company of family, we laughed about just those things and realized together we were letting off some tension. And humor was a safety valve my mother would have used herself.

So, that which I have greatly feared—and greatly expected, and even greatly prayed for has come upon me. And upon my family. My mother, thank God, passed gently into that sweet night. She had her rosary, a tape playing softly, her scapular (Thank God one was found for her!) in place. She was ready. We, her family, were ready too.

That we cried—that we will continue to cry—does not mean we were unprepared. I think, even as I write this, that this experience must be played out fully. Even the nasty casket selection process, the choices, the plans, the hassles in getting people here, everything. We will have to experience it, knowing that it is, after all, a part of life. Whether it's birth, marriage, divorce, or death, it is all part of the cycle of life.

My mother, God bless her, is no longer here to suffer or squeak out her life in pathetic little doses of reality. She is on the other side; the passage, though long, was not physically painful. The parting will extend over the next several days. Her family will mourn and laugh and go about the business of living and preparing her send-off.

Considering the angst the last several months have created for me, now I will probably feel these events are somewhat anticlimactic. I know as I write this "essay," it seems devoid of true emotion and the "heart" many of my other accounts have held. No matter. It is just an account of this day, the day my mother died. There are two more days before the funeral. More people to greet, more tears to shed. I think I will try to welcome what lies ahead now, and let myself experience this as I should.

Maybe one way would be to stop typing, and start talking—to my mother. Finally she is in a place where I can do that.

The universality, coupled with the uniqueness of losing a loved one, makes this final passage a brain-jarring one. We naturally console each other, compare heartbreaking stories and shared sorrows. The send-offs we plan supposedly celebrate the life that's been lost; the scriptures read remind us of the new life found. Yet sooner or later family and friends disperse, the black clothes are put away, and we are each left with our own thoughts, memories and emotions. We waver between numbness and searing pain, depression and joy. It's a ride I would never want to take alone, even though ultimately we must.

After waiting so long for my mother to die, I found myself both numb and raw-edged. The grieving process had been so drawn out, that when the actual "event" occurred it was as if I'd been drained of emotion. But that was only for a time. For the finality of my mother's passing away was all too real.

Finally a Funeral
Essay: November 21, 2003

Countless clichés come to mind as I ponder the reality of my mother's death and today's funeral. It doesn't seem real. It is really a blessing. She's in a better place. It's part of life.

Some friends had told me I might escape some grieving, as I have actually been grieving for two years now. I have to say I am not sure that is true. The tears came and come again. The loss is surreal, as she was lost to me for so long. But now of course I have to face the fact that I will not see her again, not touch her hand, not hear her voice. Not until some day when I will join her in heaven. My mother is dead.

I am grateful and relieved that my faith in God and belief in the hereafter makes her passing not only bearable, but truly a relief. That she *is* in a better place is a truth I cling to for comfort now. That she was after all ninety years old and "we all have to go sometime" is another reality I can accept as well.

Her funeral was today, and we got through it. I decided to read the personal essay* I had written back in August of 2002 about the lessons I've learned from her. I was nervous, but glad in a way to express my offbeat tribute for all that my mother taught me.

Oddly, I can't seem to write anymore now. Maybe I am too tired. I know there are experiences from this day that I want to record and reflect on. For one thing, I want to write about what my uncle Joe told me about my mother—stories I had never heard before.

That her life was so rich and meaningful to so many

people makes me sad and proud at the same time. My mother was a pretty remarkable woman, and I have missed her, will miss her. I hope I will soon feel a spiritual connection that I have been lacking these two years.

For now, enough of this. I will write more at another time. Maybe I need to let it all rest.

* The essay, "Things I Learned from My Mother" is included at the end of this book.

I remember, when my father-in-law died a few years earlier, noticing something I thought rather profound as I left the hospital. There were birds flitting in a nearby bush, people walking, going about their business. In other words, it was as if his passing had only happened in that room inside and only touched those gathered there. But of course the ripples spread and would spread further as more people learned of his passing.

Now too, with my mother's seemingly long overdue passing, her family was at last facing life without her. We had walked a difficult road, and now at its turn there were starts and stumbles. I continued to write when I'd visit my dad—our lives now minus my mother.

Down in the Dumps
Essay: December 30, 2003

Visiting my dad today had a different tone to it than any visit I've had before. Even as I say this though, I now think of how it was the same in so many respects. So which was it? Different *and* the same. The sameness stemmed from the usual things we did: going out to dinner, watching TV, and yes, his telling me he was feeling "down in the dumps." Another thing that was the same was how I, ever the cheerleader, tried to assure him that this was only natural. "Not to worry."

What was decidedly different of course was that there was no visit to Mom at the nursing home. Since she had passed away last month, this was my first visit back to see my dad. Not needing to take that heart-wrenching visit to see my mother was a blessing, an old routine I didn't miss.

My dad and I sat in his sun porch, the sky clouded over in heavy grayness. He made small talk as I tried even harder to push our conversation along. Among the few Christmas gifts I'd brought for him was a framed picture of my mother a few years ago as she decorated her small Christmas tree. I wondered how he'd like it, a little afraid I'd push the emotional buttons too strongly and create more sadness in him. I talked a lot, explaining the picture, attempting to soften the pain of seeing her as she had been. (This photo appears in the photographs section.)

His reaction was sweet. He seemed to take it well, even asking if I'd mind if he gave it to the Hospice nurse who still visited him regularly. I knew why he wanted to do that, since he had explained to me several days before that this person had shown him a picture of my mother while she was at the home. My dad didn't like it because Mom was too thin and looked unwell. I knew Dad wanted his new friend to see my mom as he always wanted to see her—happy and robust and full of life. I told him I'd make another copy for him to give to her, but he was to keep this one for himself.

Later I saw him looking at the picture, a moving vision of a man missing his wife. I wondered if he was longing to join her, as he admitted he feels sort of useless now. At eighty-eight, in poor health himself, it is hard for him to find purpose and drive for living. I worry that his currently slipping mood may lead to greater depths of depression.

But for now, today, he seems okay. We laugh together at a silly sitcom. Before that we'd enjoyed a meal of fish and chips, where I noticed with relief he still has a good appetite. Earlier he had been looking out the back door, commenting on the darkness of the sky. Craning his head, he noticed, "The clouds are really dark, but there's blue sky over there."

"Like life," I remarked. To his quizzical look I expanded, "It's like life, isn't it? There can be darkness, heavy clouds, but then there's blue sky and sunlight somewhere waiting to come out." He smiled. "Remember that," I said simply.

He smiled again, and I knew he would try. We all have to try to remember that. This visit was our first one without my mother, and the emptiness cannot be ignored. Yet there's always the promise of silver linings and better times. Even sweet memories can fill those empty places in our hearts.

I told my dad that I'd felt a sweet connection to my

mother the other day when I was holding my five-month-old granddaughter while she visited at my house. On my sliding glass door I had a few crocheted snowflakes my mother had made years ago. Attached with small suction cups, they hung prettily at the window, catching little Sophie's eye. I held her close enough so she could touch one, and her tiny fingers swatted at it, causing it to swing. She even tried to lift it, focused on the effort.

As I looked at her little face, her eyes fixed on the snowflake, I felt a tightness in my throat. I looked beyond her to the outside, and skyward above the trees. I sensed my mother looking on from heaven smiling with amusement as the great-granddaughter she hadn't met was reaching out to her handiwork. It was then I introduced them, the spiritual connection quite real, though bittersweet.

Connections. In life, beyond death. Of necessity it's a human quest that cannot be denied. Today I connected to my dad in ordinary, routine ways. And we both knew my mother, though absent, was still there with us. Perhaps in the gray clouds, maybe in the wind that swatted our faces as we dove into the restaurant. Maybe mostly in the laugh we shared later while watching TV. No matter, as long as she was there.

Seeing her husband "down in the dumps," maybe she can somehow pull him up. Maybe through her smile, frozen in the photograph. A smile from better times promising the connections we still seek.

The following day my dad and I visited the cemetery together. Emotionally, I found it devoid of connections. The gravesite still had the turned-over earth, no grass, with sunken soil marking the recent invasion. We stood awkwardly outside, the chilly breeze hitting us in the eyes. We didn't stay long.

We drove down to the beach then and watched the seagulls cry over unseen treasures. As we sat in the car, I knew that he and my mom used to come there often. We didn't speak much, and again we didn't stay long.

The last part of our visit was at his senior center, where I enjoyed talking to some of his friends and a few of our relatives who hang out there as well. It was less painful to leave him there among friends and family instead of leaving him alone at home.

As I drove to my own house later, I reviewed the visit in my mind as I usually do. Suddenly I was aware of a missing piece. *I wasn't crying.* For the last two years, as I zoomed along the highway after each visit, every ride home had included blurry vision from my tears. There were no tears today, and I realized then that the visit had been a better one than I might have expected.

Despite my mother's death and my father's depression, it was a better visit. Seems somehow distressing to come to that conclusion, but there it is. Better times may not have to be so good. Just good enough.

Coffee at the Cemetery
Essay: January 24, 2004

Brushing the snow off the flat stone marker at the cemetery struck me as something you might see someone do in a movie. But I did it anyway. I had driven up the long hill, passing many upright headstones to the area of flat ones. I finally pulled up to what I'd estimated was my mother's gravesite.

My dad sat without speaking, sipping a too-hot coffee we had just purchased at a nearby drive-through doughnut shop. I had been the one to suggest we could bring the coffee with us on this brutally cold January afternoon and just pay Mom a little visit.

"Not that she's really there," I added quickly, as I attempted to chase away the gloomy thoughts that pull at my brain and leaden my heart. I can't bear to think of my mom there under the cold dark ground. Happily, as a faithful Christian, I can lift my eyes and know instead that she is in heaven. Still, visiting a loved one's gravesite seems "the thing to do," so there we were.

As cold as it was, I had first intended to sit in the car with my dad, sipping our coffee and letting conversation rise or fall as the spirit led us. I was as surprised as he was when I suddenly said, "Stay here, I'm going outside." And with that I gave my scarf another twist around my neck and ventured out onto the snow-covered ground, the wind blustering its way up the hill and catching my breath before it left my throat.

As I said, I had parked my car in front of a section of earth where I thought my mother's spot was. Now I saw I had overshot it by a few feet. It was while straining to see the flat stones, that I did see the pinkish hue that identified her stone to me. That's when I began to brush the snow away, clearing the picture of the Blessed Mother, and revealing my mother's name. The date of her death had yet to be etched in, her death having been just two months ago. I noticed that the ground, though hard and heavily dusted with snow, still had that fresh grave look to it as well.

In time I allowed myself to look over the length of it. More slowly still I let myself talk aloud to my mother. I began as I had said to my father, "I know you're not really in there now." Then it came in a rush: the reality of missing her. For a moment I wanted to dash back to the car to get the pictures I had of my granddaughter, the baby my mother had never seen. I resisted, though barely.

Instead, I told my mom those things I was feeling, the tears misting my eyes. Despite the spiritual connections and the healing process and all that other stuff that has been happening, I was of course standing at my mother's grave. The wind was whipping the dry snow around the stone again, and I knew in a few days an upcoming storm would cover it completely.

I ended my visit saying a "Hail Mary" and commenting to my mom that she had a lovely spot here on the hill overlooking Narragansett Bay. I wondered if it mattered, given her post in heaven, but I knew she and my dad had picked this spot many years earlier. That did make the view seem more important I supposed.

Now, with my toes going numb, I turned away and headed back to the car.

Climbing inside, I told my dad we had passed the site a bit, so I backed the car up and gave him a minute to privately commune with his wife of sixty-three years. I started up the car then and pulled away, being careful of the deep ruts along the edge of the road. I remarked to my dad that there were still many

Christmas decorations throughout the cemetery. A strange mix of joy and sorrow.

Our coffee had grown cold as we headed back to the little house only a mile away. As we went inside, still chilled from the outdoors, I realized my mother was more present here than she was at the gravesite. It was a comforting thought really, but I knew the process of saying good-bye to my mother wasn't over by a long shot.

My dad and I finished the dregs of our cold coffee. He dozed off with the TV on as I sat in my mother's chair and missed her profoundly. Later that evening, alone in my old bedroom, I pulled out the pictures of my granddaughter and showed them to my mother.

Though tears were running from my eyes, I believe we both smiled.

So, This Is It
Essay: February 28, 2004

This afternoon I sat in my mother's cushioned rocking chair, staring out the window onto her backyard. Of course the trees were now devoid of leaves, and although it was an unusually warm day, the winter shades of gray and brown reflected an undeniable bleakness.

I noticed the large plaster statue of the Blessed Mother stood as it always had, surrounded by plant pots and plastic animals. A sheep lay on its side, and every pot held tangled brown masses of weeds and dead flowers. It was a mess. If my mother were alive, I mused, she'd likely have a fit.

But of course, she is dead.

I sighed, and turned my eyes back to my father who sat opposite the windows on a stained but comfortable loveseat. It was a Lazy-Boy recliner, and years ago he had purchased it himself to enjoy in the sun porch. He would sit with his legs up and listen to my mother talk in ways only a man who's been married for over six decades can listen to his wife. His hearing loss probably helped.

Now he sat, asleep, shallow breathing beating an eerie rhythm as his chest moved up and down. His head was bent and his big hands were clasped over his slight paunch. I wondered if he was dreaming of better times, but I turned my attention back to the window. I sighed again.

This is the view my mother had for all those years she lived here in this little house. When I'd visit, I too would sit on the loveseat, sharing confidences and getting advice. Now, as I looked out on the yard, I tried to see it through my mother's eyes. Just past the maple tree, my brother's yard met theirs, and with little obstruction she could see his house. I knew she noticed their comings and goings as his side door was in plain view.

I knew she watched the birds and worried when a cat crept across the lawn. And I know she gazed on the statue of Mary and whispered prayers. Sitting in her chair today, I saw it all and missed her. I closed my eyes and let the warm sun touch my face, trying to nap as my dad so comfortably did. No luck there. Too many thoughts, too many aches.

My father woke up, looking almost embarrassed he had slept so long. Remembering I was there to visit him, he asked me what I wanted to do for the rest of the afternoon. I tossed the question back to him, but he had no suggestions.

Without saying it, we realized we were at a loss here. We had done the lunch thing together, and this resting at home was fine. Of course what was missing was the routine visit to see my mother at the nursing home. We had done it for two years, and in that time had at least gotten over the emptiness of not having her there at the house.

As I sat in her chair I realized *she* hadn't sat there in over two years. She hadn't seen her yard as the seasons changed them. She had never seen the new windows my dad had put in to cut down on the draftiness. She hadn't been there in a very long time.

"Do you want to go get some coffee?" I suggested to my father. "Then we could go to the cemetery." This last bit I held out tentatively. We had done that the last time I came to visit, and I knew it had gone okay. And I knew I wanted to go there, even for just a little while.

"Good idea," he said as if I had just suggested going to see a good movie.

Fifteen minutes later, we were driving up the cemetery road, taking the hot coffee along for the ride.

"At least we don't have to visit her at the nursing home," my dad said.

"Yeah, you're right," I replied, realizing the implied truth of that simple exchange was that being dead was better than being in a home—or at least it was better for us, her family.

Yet, we knew it had to be better for her too. Visions of her sitting with her head on the table or complaining, "I want to go home," came uninvited into my mind.

Well, she was home now.

And this is it, I thought. This will be the way the visits will go now. Dad and I will do the lunch thing, visit the cemetery, and maybe go out for dinner at that place by the water. It's a little expensive, but several visits ago I'd concluded it was worth it. I don't see him that often. We can't do it every week. And who knew how many more times we could do it anyway? So it was added to our routine.

And now the cemetery visit has taken the place of the nursing home visit. As I stood by the gravesite, I felt, as I had before, strangely disconnected, unsure of what to do or what to say or even how to pray. Looking down at the rough earth, I wondered when there'd be grass there instead of the ugly brown dirt that only reminded us how recently she'd been buried. But then it's only been three months, and grass can't grow in winter.

What possessed me to pick up a rock and put it in my pocket? I don't know. It's a strange memento, a simple connection to my mother's gravesite. I knew I would put it on my kitchen windowsill where I could see it everyday.

I guess this is how my visits will go now. The saga of the nursing home has ended. My grieving can now take a new turn. I realized this morning before I started off for my dad's house that I was not feeling the dread I had for years. Maybe that is the best I can experience now, as these visits become whatever they must become.

Now that my mother is gone.

My writing about my mother continued sporadically after her passing away. Though I still visited my father of course, the need to record those personal events ebbed, at least a bit. Within my own daily life, I found myself connected to my mom in many ways, and of these I would sometimes write. I offer two of those essays here. I'll then add a couple more I'd referred to earlier in this book. Then I think it is time to stop—stop adding essays, though maybe not stop writing them. And of course, I'll never stop missing my mother.

With Sympathy
Essay: October 19, 2004

My mother's birthday was the day before yesterday. She would have turned ninety-one. Then again, it's still incredible to me that she lived to see ninety. In just one month it will be a year that she passed away—just before Thanksgiving last year.

While I walked to church on her birthday, I wondered if she was having a birthday party up in heaven. I hoped so as she really didn't get to have one the last two years of her life. Trapped in a mind that was failing her, she was hardly aware of what day it was; never mind acknowledging her birthday.

Through the last several years I sometimes saw her on that day, sometimes not. I know that last year I opted to visit my new granddaughter instead of traveling the two hours to sit at the nursing home with my mother as she turned ninety. I learned later that no one else in the family decided to celebrate the day—not as we used to anyway. She wasn't sure what day it was, soon forgot who had just visited, and in other ways was distant from us, even from herself.

That's why I was thinking of sympathy cards. At first I thought briefly of looking at birthday cards, just as some twisted exercise in getting in touch with my feelings. I always sent her a card at least, and chose the verse well. But there was no point in torturing myself that way this year. What about a sympathy card? Oh sure, no torture there.

The collection of cards I received after my mother's death still lies in my dresser drawer. Held fast with an elastic band, the bulging pile offers comfort and sympathy on the loss of my mother. Thing is, I'd already lost her. And no one sent me a card two years ago.

No one sent a card when she stopped talking to me on the phone. There was no card in the mail when she began to forget who I was. When she stopped asking how my children were, I knew I had lost my mother. But Hallmark apparently doesn't make a condolence card for *lost lives*—only death.

So now she is dead. I still get kind form letters from Hospice. They assure me the grieving process is long and complex. They tell me to be prepared for unexpected reminders of my loved one—and unexpected waves of fresh grief as the loss is revisited. This I know is true.

Yet what I can't seem to wrap my head around is the long good-bye. The process that took her away from me in endless bits and pieces. When I said my real good-bye to my mother, she was barely herself. Yet she lived over a year longer, and my connection to her grew fainter as those months wore on. Writing about that torturous passage gives me some closure I suppose. I documented well each visit to the nursing home, each heartache as I watched her slip further and further away.

More painful still were those times when she seemed more lucid. There were visits when she appeared more connected, and this had its own horror for me as I wondered how lonely she must feel or how frightened.

"It's a blessing." was the sentiment passed around the funeral home when she finally passed away. There was no denying that "she's better off" now. Her suffering is over.

But I still miss my mother.

Today at the mall I saw a little old lady. Barely five feet tall, her face was crinkly, her short hair held just the right mixture of gray. Her eyes held a hint of confusion, but I could see kindness in them as she smiled back at me. (I had to smile at her because I had first *stared* at her.) She reminded me of my mother. I wanted to go up to her and ask how old she was and tell her she made me think of my mother.

Fortunately, accosting strangers at the mall is something I don't do, so I let it pass. Still, the brief exchange brought home to me once again how much my mother is always on my mind. Later when I saw a bird trying to find shelter from the wind, I again thought of my mother and how she loved birds. Still later, I wrote a few checks out to charities and remembered how my mother would always stuff a couple of dollar bills in an envelope and send them off to her favorite causes.

I remember my mother. Not as the wasting away woman who had her head down on the table at the nursing home.

Instead I strive to remember her as the loving, caring mom with strong faith and a keen sense of humor.

Yes, I miss my mother. It's been nearly a year. She hardly had an "untimely death," but I still miss her. And no, Hallmark doesn't have a card to offer sympathy for such a long and sad good-bye. So much for closure.

Mother's Day
Essay: May 13, 2005

I spent Mother's Day with my daughter and granddaughter. It was great. But I missed my mother. She has been dead for nearly a year and a half, and I still feel the loss.

She was lost to me for years before her death due to dementia. I close my eyes sometimes to focus my memory on her face and her voice. I remember garbled messages left on our answering machine, and I wish I could hear them again. I remember her smile or the touch of her hand and I miss her. She was ninety when she died, I in my mid-fifties—neither of us seemingly in need of mothering. Yet I still feel a hole in my life where my mother used to be.

How many books have been written about the mother-daughter bond? Too many I'd suspect. But now that my tie to my own mother has been supposedly severed by her passing, I see that the mystery of what holds us to our moms is pretty powerful stuff.

I looked at my daughter during our Mother's Day visit

and saw the future as she tended to her child. I saw the past too as I considered how my mother must have thought the same thoughts I did as I watched "my little girl" with her little girl.

I knew somehow there was a multigenerational link, and even a connection beyond the perimeters of this life. My mother may be gone, but she is always with me. I knew as she was suffering through her last two years in a nursing home, she was then at a place I couldn't find her. She would barely remember when I'd last been to see her, or even at times what was my name. Now that she has passed on, I sense we are somehow closer than we were. My faith in God allows me to picture her in heaven, her spirit at last free. She is more accessible in a way.

I look back at the years before the nursing home, the years when she was truly my mom. Even as an adult I could call her, hear her advice or ask for her prayers. Those are the contacts I really miss. That they were pulled away from me gradually doesn't seem to ease the pain of losing them.

I can see her all around me in every crocheted doily in my house, in every dish that had been hers, even in the jacket that I wear—I took it from her closet after she died. When I put it on, it's like she's hugging me. She is all around me. Her favorite prayer book sits on my bedroom lamp table, and her favorite recipe is lodged in my memory. How can I miss my mother?

Mother's Day perhaps should have found me at her gravesite, a pot of spring flowers ready to place beside her stone. Instead I chose to spend it embracing the life that is my daughter and the even brighter life that is my granddaughter. I know my mother would approve. And I know, really know in my heart, that my mother knows I miss her.

Sometimes I wonder if she misses me. In truth, wondering how she thought of me through those tormenting two years troubles me still. I needed to believe she was in a stage of "*un*knowing," but at times the clarity of her mind and the apparent emotions were unsettling. No matter—those days are past. No use dwelling on them. If she suffered, I feel badly of course. But I suffered too.

I was missing my mother, robbed of who she was. I had to say good-bye long before she truly left. And so I guess every Mother's Day will prompt me to reflect on the relationship I had with my mom. It will force me to look back and experience the feelings again. It is all testimony to the unending relationship we have with our mothers. And for that I suppose I should be grateful. I imagine though, that I will always have a sense of loss when I think of my mother.

Until I too pass on and join her. During her last months she would say: "I want to go home to my mother." I thought then, and I believe now, that she knew exactly what she was saying. Her mother, long dead, was probably a welcoming sight for my mom as she passed on. It must have been a comfort really.

So, yeah, Happy Mother's Day, Mom. I hope you are happy where you are, and know that you are always in my heart. Still.

Epilogue

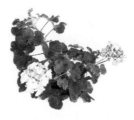

The following essay is the one I read at my mother's funeral. Though written years before and not intended to be shared in that way, it became an act of closure for me at that time.

Things My Mother Taught Me
Written August 4, 2002
Read at her funeral November 21, 2003

I was at a restaurant not long ago and I had to use the bathroom, really bad. I rushed into the stall and for half a second I almost just sat myself down to get on with business. But I didn't. I took the time to cover the toilet seat with toilet paper. This happening is not insignificant, because I knew in that short passage of time that the action I was taking was a direct result of what my mother had taught me: "You cover toilet seats in public places because God only knows what germs you might pick up if you don't."

That sure knowledge is obviously so ingrained in me that I automatically responded to it. It made me consider what else do I do automatically because I learned from my mother these basic rules of life. On reflection, all kinds of things come to mind from "Always cook pork till it's cooked through" to "Never miss Mass on Sunday unless you're really sick." Of course there's a corollary rule to that last one: "If you do miss Mass you can't go out anywhere else that day." This also applies to missing school, by the way, and this one I follow religiously—more religiously than the church one I'm afraid. But let's move on . . .

My mother had some tried and true sayings that she did her best to have me absorb. One of my all-time favorites was "Why buy the cow if the milk is free?" This refers of course to the moral and ethical question of premarital sex. Through my teen years I always knew talking about sex wasn't something she felt comfortable with, but I always knew firmly where she stood on those kinds of issues.

Another classic lesson my mother taught me was "If your husband is earning $10,000 and you're spending $11,000, you're going to be poor. But if he's earning $10,000 and you're spending $9,000, your family will be all set." Nowhere in that scenario did she ever suggest the wife could go out and earn that lousy extra grand herself and thereby be able to spend as she might wish. The message was clear and I saw her live it every day of her sixty-plus years of married life.

I learned that you darn socks, you don't just throw them out. Thanks to my mom, I know that you really don't need that many pairs of shoes, and you should try not to buy *anything* if it's not on sale. She taught me to work for what you need, not for what you want. I grew up hearing that "A penny saved is a penny earned" and you waited patiently for those pennies to add up. *Then* you could make that purchase. I can remember licking S&H Green Stamps and, in a grand conspiracy, discovering we finally had enough for those lamps or that tray table.

My mother had the questionable distinction in the family of being a "Pick-a-Fighter." She earned this title by her willingness to call any insurance agency, any bill collector, or even the town hall for any member of our very extended family who was having a problem. I learned not to accept things if they seemed unjust and to stand up for what was right.

My mother had no use for people who put on airs and thought they were better than other people. Clothes and cars were so much worldly trappings and provided no measurement of a person's character. She was a soft touch for any charity and for years would slip a dollar or two into any envelope that came her way. She always felt that the thank you notes sent to her by this charity or that cause were personal and sincere. I quickly gave up trying to explain the ease at which these notes were computer-generated. Instead I let her teach me the lesson of giving without expecting a return.

I learned how to cook from my mother, although my own family now teases me that I rarely have a recipe I can share. I learned that you make Portuguese roast meat by first pouring vinegar into the roasting pan until the liquid meets around the edges. And I can remember my mom telling me that if there weren't clam boils in heaven already, she'd start cooking them.

I know without a doubt that the most important thing my mother taught me was to have faith in God. I remember the countless rosaries prayed, the treks through chapels and churches. I can even remember her wearing brown for weeks in tribute to Our Lady of Mount Carmel as part of a novena or prayer for her intercession. I remember my mother reading from her black imitation-leather prayer book, with many pages soiled from constant use as she prayed to the Holy Spirit for guidance and comfort.

I guess I'd have to say I learned perseverance from my mother. For years she was ill, having many trips to the hospital for one thing or the other. Often it seemed she was sent to share and talk and pray for whatever roommate she might have. She endured tests and treatments and operations, and yet she moved on to the next trial with unwavering faith.

She was scared at times and known to complain about this pain or that, and I suppose I learned that's okay too. Each of us is only human after all. As a child I experienced that special treatment she'd provide when I was sick. Fresh sheets on *her* bed with the cool white bedspread, ginger ale and saltines on the bedside table, and I was set up comfortably for the day. All grown up, with children of my own, I tried to duplicate that example of tender loving care. Maybe the lesson was sweet though impractical: someone will take care of you when you're sick.

Toward the end of my mother's life her family (me included of course), became unable to take care of her. Not without some guilt and much sadness did we admit her to a nursing home. Early in her stay I spoke with her about getting ready to go to heaven. She seemed resolved to pass over without a fight. That day while visiting, I had the unique and dreaded blessing of saying good-bye to my mother. I thanked her for all the things she taught me and singled out the faith as the gift I will always treasure the most. With a catch in my voice I expressed to her my fear that I may not have succeeded in passing that on to my own children. Her rueful smile made me take courage that those things we teach our children may not always seem learned.

As I spoke with her that day I asked her if she knew much about dying. When she said she didn't, I told her what I knew from reading books—about passing through tunnels and bright light, and people you love greeting you from the other side. It occurred to me in that bittersweet conversation that as my mother had taught me the facts of life, here was I trying to teach her some facts of death.

That farewell was a strange one, mostly because she didn't die. I had many visits after that one, but truly as her mind and memory deteriorated, another opportunity for such an exchange no longer existed. I realized I had received a special gift, a chance to tell my mother how I loved her and treasured all those life lessons.

One more gift I should mention is her sense of humor, which could be silly or cynical, but always a good lesson in how to deal with life's little foibles. I know she'd get a kick out of knowing I think of her whenever I cover a toilet seat—as long as I also remember her in every prayer and every flower bed and every good thing that is my life.

As I write this, my mom is still alive, but somehow

already gone from us. Her memory loss is severe, yet thankfully she still remembers her family. Conversations tend to be shallow and one-sided. The time spent together today will be long forgotten tomorrow. Ah, one last lesson, sad and sweet: "Live in the moment, treasure time spent with those you love." Another thing I learned from my mother.

Thanks, Mom.

Postscript 11/16/02
(Note: The following additions to this essay were not read at her funeral)

My last visit with my mother found her "stuck" in a recurring statement, almost a chant. With her head resting on the table, she would pick it up occasionally to say, "I want to go home, I want to go home, I want to go home to my mother." Finally I asked her what home she was talking about. She said, without hesitation, "I'm talking about heaven."

I left her that day feeling as sad as I've ever felt. For all she's taught me, I had no answer for what to do when God's way is so seemingly at odds with our own. On second thought, I did have an answer. I told her to ask the Lord about all that. I told her to pray. Thanks again, Mom, for the lesson that carries us best through this life—and possibly into the next: pray and trust in God. *Period.*

Postscript 1/6/03

I saw my mother alive for possibly the last time last Sunday. A brief holiday visit with at least one important mission. I got to tell my mother that my daughter is pregnant. In truth she was at first confused, asking if Jen was getting married. When I patiently explained she already was married and was now expecting a baby, my mother of eighty-nine years clapped her hands and said, "Oh goodie!" I know I will wish I could ask her advice on becoming a grandmother; I know she would have things to teach me. As she is slipping now into the next life, I know I will have to rely on those things she's already taught me. For all of those things I remain grateful—and confident that the lessons will not be lost.

This next essay relates to my introduction where I mention my mother "losing her marbles." I still do have that bag, and yes, this essay is attached to it.

Mom's Marbles
Written February 20, 2003

Years ago my mother told me she was *not* "losing her marbles" and she was angry that the people around her seemed to think she was. It was a conversation started, as many were back then, by her relating to me what she had foolishly done or forgotten to do. In her lapses, my dad or my brother or maybe her sister would voice their concern and she would get mad. "I'm *not* losing my marbles," she would insist to me.

I would reassure her, "I'm sure you still have all your marbles, Mom. Don't worry." It was easy to tell her not to worry since *I* was doing that, along with the rest of the family. Still, as a gesture of support, I found a cute bag of marbles at a toy store and mailed them to her. I included a note that said, "The next time you feel like someone is saying you're losing your marbles, just show them these!" Typically she got quite a kick out of that, and we would laugh over the phone many times about that marble bag. I hadn't much thought about them lately.

Until tonight, when I found my mother's marbles.

Back from visiting her in the home, I was raiding the cracker cabinet for a snack. When I visit, I stay overnight with my dad, and although graham crackers and milk were my mom's and my favorite bedtime snack, I offered to get some for him.

He declined, but I padded into the kitchen to get myself a little something.

And there in the corner of the cabinet was the marble bag. I had to smile and knew right then I had to have them. Knowing my dad had recently told me, "Take whatever you want," I knew he'd be okay with this, but I felt I should ask anyway.

"Dad, can I take these?" I asked, showing him the small net bag with about five or six large marbles. He looked dubiously at what lay in my hand but answered, "Sure."

Although he didn't ask, I felt a need to explain, at least in part. "Mom and I had a silly joke going about these marbles," was all I said. He smiled, said nothing, and I added, "I'd like to have them—for sentimental reasons."

So now they're mine.

As I look at them, the silly conversations come back to me, as does the bittersweet realization that my efforts at supporting my mother were ultimately unsuccessful. I guess you'd have to say she eventually lost her marbles. She is in a home, has been for well over a year because she can't take care of herself, forgetting things almost right away.

I wonder if I brought the marbles in to show her when I visit again if she would be able to remember what they were about. Because I doubt it, I know I won't even try. Somehow it would be cruel. The marbles were supposed to be a comfort, an assurance that all was not lost, that she could maintain her mental acuity and stay intact.

She was afraid of "losing her marbles." I know that, knew it even back then, and my joking efforts were an attempt to reassure both of us that she was okay. But of course she wasn't, and it soon became apparent that a little bag of glass marbles could not stop the loss she was experiencing.

But now I have the bag, and what am I going to do with them? Common sense tells me to tuck them away somewhere in my house, but with a note attached. For someday someone may come across them and wonder why on earth I would have saved them.

Someday I may come across them and wonder the same thing. That I might not remember is the scenario that frightens me the most. That I might "lose my marbles" is a fear that sadly haunts me as it would anyone whose parent has a severe memory loss.

So, let this little story be "the note," with one addition:

"I am saving this silly little bag of marbles to remind myself that my mother insisted she was *not* losing hers; and I, her daughter, made her laugh even as I supported her. *Please, someone, do that for me.*"

Closing Thoughts

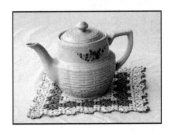

This collection of journal entries and essays took more than six years to compile and edit—I couldn't even start the process until my mother had been gone over two years. (Somehow sobbing as I sat at my computer cut down on the efficiency of my task.) Many years later, the sobbing was less frequent, though the memories were made fresh. My father went on to join my mother when he died in 2007. Finally getting this account together seemed a way to grieve him too, even as I honor both their memories.

I began this project by saying writing saves things. And yes, I do want to save this experience—not just for myself, but also for others. Through the years writing has played an important role for me. A gift from God to help me cope with reality, it has provided me with a sounding board and a record of His grace. Beyond dealing with the death of loved ones, there's been my mother's dementia, my son's divorce, my father's depression, and other relationship issues. All of these life experiences have found a path to peace through my writing. Despite my dreadful humanness, God provided what I needed to see me through each circumstance.

Writing was a big part, but not everything of course.

As each of us struggles with our own challenges, those things that define our personal "faith journey," we need to be aware of those "life-preservers" God throws our way. It might be having coffee with a friend, the kind of friend you can cry with and share your deepest fears. For some people, meditation keeps them grounded, for others soft music can settle frayed nerves. Still others find solace in a bag of M&Ms. (Do be careful of "stress-eating" though; that's a curse, not a blessing!) Better choices would be to schedule a day's "retreat" or a massage if that helps you relax. It's best to find some healthy ways to redirect any negative energy into that positive, life-affirming state of mind that eludes us during times of personal crisis.

There are certain truths in life that help if we hang onto them. (At times we'll feel we're clinging by our fingernails!) Consider finding and memorizing special Bible passages or other quotations that particularly inspire or console you. (I love Psalm 91–what a comforting "contract" with God.) Just knowing "This too shall pass" can be enough to snap us back into a broader perspective, thus saving us from extended grief.

But never deny the grieving process its due.

Suppressing our emotions, even fearing them is not helpful. Instead, we should strive to acknowledge and understand them. Joining a support group might be a way for some people to process their emotions. Whatever the avenue, we need to remind ourselves that we are okay. We may feel guilty, we might be "selfish," but we should realize that we must be our own best friends. Taking care of ourselves is not a bad thing; it's a good thing. For me, just having my fleece robe run through the clothes dryer for a few minutes before I climb into it can make me feel pampered.

And yes, we all need mothering–even if unforeseen circumstances force us to search for it with heavy hearts.

It is my hope that sharing this account, this memorial to my mother's last two years, will resonate with those who suffer similar experiences. Hopefully it will somehow draw us all closer: family, friends, and fellow wanderers through these painful passages of life.

It is my prayer that through this tiny contribution, this little bit of recorded life experience, we will all see the unwavering faithfulness of God. Throughout this book I talked about seeking the "peace that passes all understanding." Having no halo on my head, I continue to seek it.

Let me end this book by leaving the actual scripture quotation for us all to ponder. For ultimately we walk alone with our God. And we find His mercy revealed in our own lives.

"Be anxious for nothing, but in everything by prayer and supplication, with thanksgiving, let your requests be made known to God; and the peace of God, which surpasses all understanding, will guard your hearts and minds through Christ Jesus."
(Phil 4:6-8)

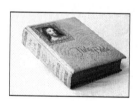

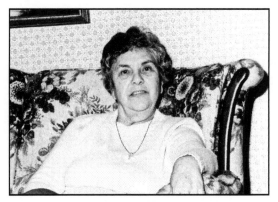

Better Days:
my mother in her sixties.

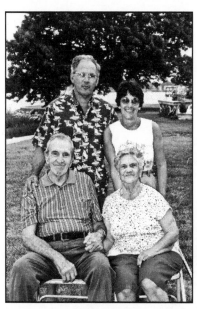

My parents, brother, and I at the Norris cottage in Mystic in 1999. We'd gather every August to celebrate Dad's birthday.

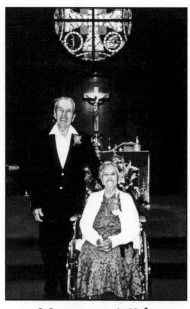

My parents' 60th anniversary, June 2000, at the altar of Holy Ghost Church in Tiverton, RI.

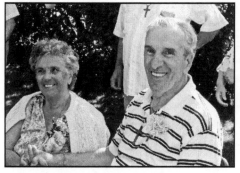

My parents hold hands at the family gathering celebrating their 49th anniversary in 1989.

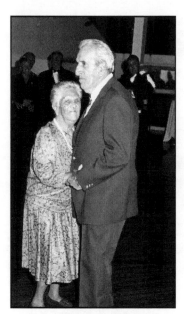

My parents at my daughter's wedding, October 1999 (later I had to remind Mom that Jen was married).

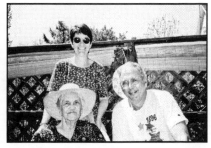

My mother, brother John, and I on our parents' deck, Mother's Day 2000.

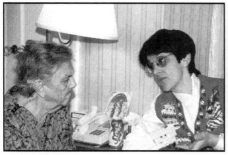

Christmas, 1999: I explain to Mom how the "picture phone" will help her (no numbers to try to remember).

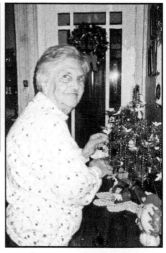

The picture I gave my dad after Mom passed away. I have a duplicate as part of my own Christmas decorations.

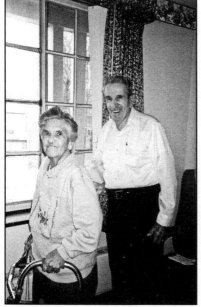

My parents in front of her room's window, 2001 (in journal entry 12/16/2001).

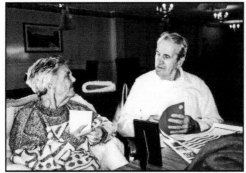

Our first Christmas at the nursing home, 2001: my parents remark on their gifts.

What a threesome: visiting in the parlor at the nursing home, 2003.

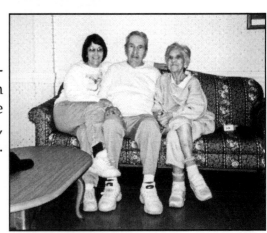

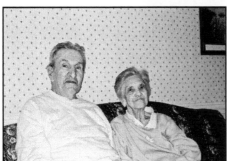

My parents snuggling together on the parlor sofa at the nursing home in 2003.

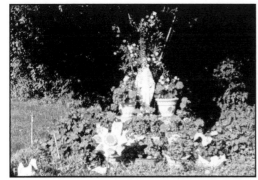

Visible from her chair: my mom's statue of the Blessed Mother in their backyard.

A backyard cook-out in 1997. This favorite snapshot sits on my desk.

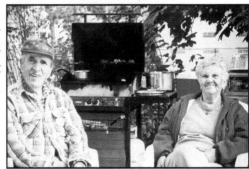

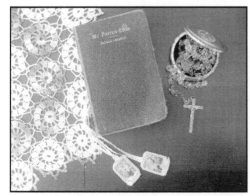

Atop one of my mother's crocheted doilies: her prayer book, wedding rosary, and an old scapular.

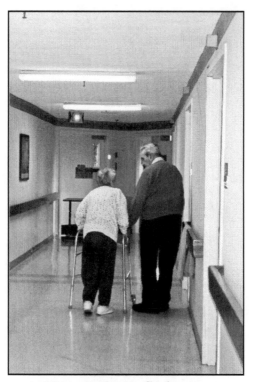

My parents at the home.
The image holds a deep
meaning for me as I see
them walking *away*.